Rapid Review of
TOXICOLOGY

Rapid Review of
TOXICOLOGY

For MBBS and postgraduate students of
Forensic Medicine and Toxicology
&
Those preparing for NEET/other PG Entrance Examinations

Tanuj Kanchan
MBBS DFM MD
Associate Professor
Department of Forensic Medicine and Toxicology
All India Institute of Medical Sciences
Jodhpur, Rajasthan, India

Forewords

Sanjeev Misra
MS MCh FRCS (Eng) FRCS (Glasgow) FICS FACS (USA) FAMS

G Pradeep Kumar
MD DFM Dip Cr Law Fellow of the Indian Academy of Forensic Medicine

JAYPEE

JAYPEE BROTHERS MEDICAL PUBLISHERS
The Health Sciences Publisher
New Delhi | London

Jaypee Brothers Medical Publishers (P) Ltd

Headquarters
EMCA House
23/23-B, Ansari Road, Daryaganj
New Delhi 110 002, India
Landline: +91-11-23272143,
+91-11-23272703
+91-11-23282021, +91-11-23245672
E-mail: jaypee@jaypeebrothers.com

Corporate Office
Jaypee Brothers Medical Publishers (P) Ltd.
4838/24, Ansari Road, Daryaganj
New Delhi 110 002, India
Phone: +91-11-43574357
Fax: +91-11-43574314
E-mail: jaypee@jaypeebrothers.com

Overseas Office
JP Medical Ltd.
83, Victoria Street, London
SW1H 0HW (UK)
Phone: +44-20 3170 8910
E-mail: info@jpmedpub.com

EU GPSR Authorised Representative
Logos Europe, 9 rue Nicolas Poussin
17000, La Rochelle, France
Phone: +33 (0) 6 67 93 73 78
E-mail: Contact@logoseurope.eu

Website: www.jaypeebrothers.com
Website: www.jaypeedigital.com

Inquiries for bulk sales may be solicited at: jaypee@jaypeebrothers.com

Rapid Review of Toxicology

First Edition: 2018, Reprint: **2026**

ISBN: 978-93-5270-131-5

Printed in India

Dedicated to

My mother Smt Suman Kanchan and father (Late) Dr TK Kanchan
for their blessings and making me what I am today

My wife, Shweta, and son, Suryaansh
for their patience, understanding and all the support throughout this endeavor

My teachers and colleagues for their continuous guidance and encouragement
and
All the students of Forensic Medicine and Toxicology
for whom, this book has come into existence.

Contributors

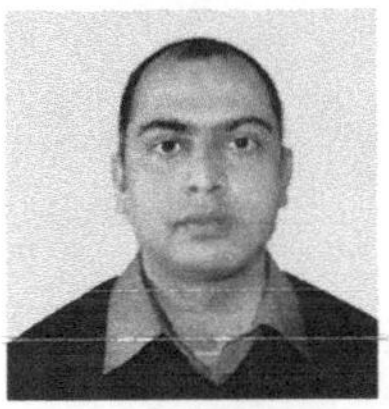

Alok Atreya MD
Assistant Professor
Department of Forensic Medicine
Nepal Medical College and Teaching Hospital
Kathmandu, Nepal
For co-authoring the chapters: Deliriants, Warfare Agents and Poison Information Center, and for contributions to the chapters: Drug Dependence and Drug Abuse

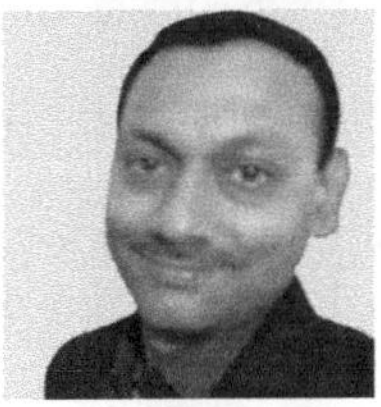

Saurabh Chattopadhyay MD
Professor and Head
Department of Forensic Medicine and Toxicology
Malda Medical College
Malda, West Bengal, India
For co-authoring the chapter: Inebriants

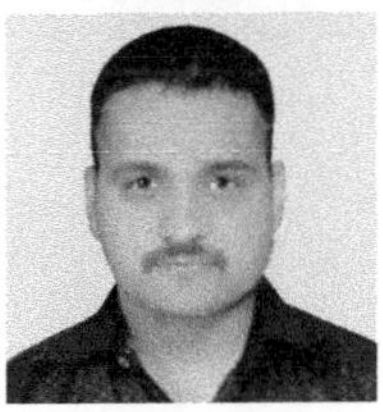

Raghvendra Singh Shekhawat MD
Assistant Professor
Department of Forensic Medicine and Toxicology
All India Institute of Medical Sciences
Jodhpur, Rajasthan, India
For co-authoring the chapter: Common Household Poisons

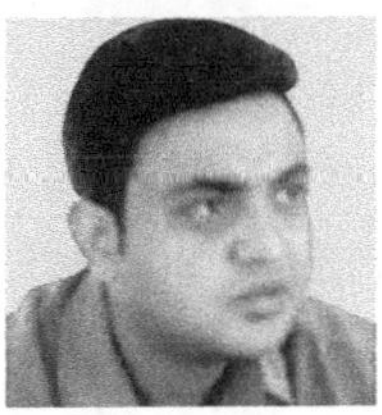

Jenash Acharya MD
Assistant Professor (Acting HOD)
Department of Forensic Medicine
Kathmandu Medical College and Teaching Hospital
Secretary
Medico-legal Society of Nepal (MeLeSoN)
Kathmandu, Nepal
For contributions to the chapter: Food Poisoning

Foreword

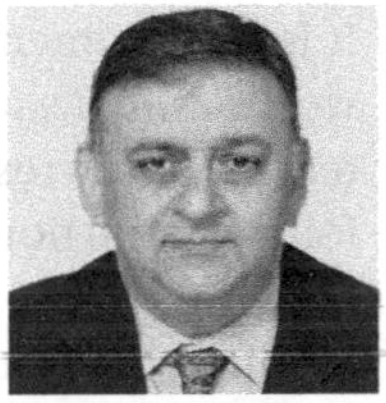

Quality textbooks and good teachers have the capability to instill in their students love and confidence for any subject, and toxicology can be no exception. I have known Dr Tanuj as one of our fine teachers and researchers at All India Institute of Medical Sciences (AIIMS), Jodhpur, Rajasthan, and the book *Rapid Review of Toxicology* is another feather in his cap.

The effort put on by the author in coming up with this novel way of presentation of text in Question-and-Answer format is commendable. Though the contents are presented in Question-and-Answer format for the students to know what is expected from them in examinations, the author has made sure that the continuity of the topics are not lost anywhere. The description in the form of flowcharts, tables and images is certainly going to help the students develop keen interest and an easy understanding of the subject. Another highlight of the book is the inclusion of Problem-based Questions, which is one of the innovative methods of teaching–learning these days. Besides, the author's endeavor to include an up-to-date information on the latest in the field of toxicology is praiseworthy. All in all, the way entire text has been presented in the book, makes it an interesting read.

The hard work put in by the author in coming up with this book is self-evident. Going through the contents of the book, *Rapid Review of Toxicology*, I am reminded of a quote by Sir Francis Bacon: "*Some books are to be tasted, others to be swallowed, and some few to be chewed and digested*". This book most certainly falls in the third category and will not only help the undergraduates and postgraduate students of forensic medicine and toxicology in better understanding of the subject, but also those preparing for NEET and other competitive postgraduate entrance examinations. I am confident that the readers will find the book useful, and author's effort will be appreciated equally by the medical students, scholars, teachers, and clinicians.

Sanjeev Misra
MS MCh FRCS (Eng) FRCS (Glasgow) FICS FACS (USA) FAMS
Professor of Surgical Oncology
Director and CEO
All India Institute of Medical Sciences
Jodhpur, Rajasthan, India

Foreword

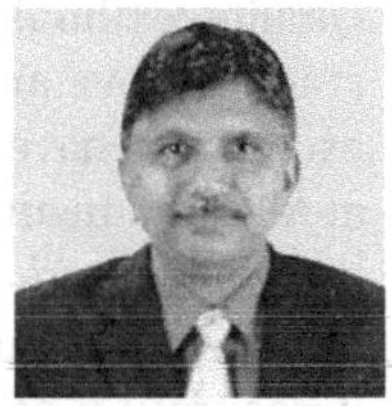

It is with immense pleasure and pride to me, to pen this foreword for the work *Rapid Review of Toxicology* scripted by Dr Tanuj Kanchan, a renowned teacher, and a research scholar par excellence, who commands a substantial followership not only in India but also across the world. I had the privilege of being closely associated with Prof Tanuj for over a decade at Kasturba Medical College, Manipal University, as a resident postgraduate and a colleague.

Toxicology is an indispensable component and an essential subject in the making of a doctor. It is not just an examination subject, but also a subject to practice and follow lifelong for every physician associated with emergency medicine. The author has done a commendable job in the narration of the subject of toxicology to stimulate and sustain the interest of the readers with lucid presentation supplemented with flowcharts, diagrams, and mnemonics wherever necessary. The author has adopted a novel method of narration of the subject, in the form of question and answer to kindle a meaningful learning habit amongst learners. The content not only fulfills the requirements of the regulatory body, but also provides adequate information to succeed in the national eligibility test essential to qualify for postgraduate admission. Dr Tanuj has toiled immensely to provide an up-to-date information in the field of toxicology, and help students achieve their goals. I strongly feel that this manual will be a very useful resource material not only to the medical professionals but also to the law enforcing agencies.

Survival of the fittest could be an apt tagline for this book, though there are several books in the market, this book will certainly leave a lasting impact on the pupils. Dr Tanuj being the recipient of the coveted good teacher at Kasturba Medical College, Mangaluru, Karnataka with his immense teaching talents will create a space of his own for this text to facilitate an effective and meaningful learning for the medical students. I am certain that the reader's inquisitiveness will be enhanced upon perusal of this text.

G Pradeep Kumar
MD DFM Dip Cr Law Fellow of the Indian Academy of Forensic Medicine
Professor, Department of Forensic Medicine
Melaka Manipal Medical College, Manipal Campus
Former Professor and Head, Department of Forensic Medicine
Kasturba Medical College, Manipal
Former Dean, Kasturba Medical College, Manipal University, Manipal
Formerly Director, Department of Quality & Compliance, Manipal University
Manipal, Karnataka, India

Preface

Toxicology is a vast subject that is first introduced to the undergraduate students of medicine in the subject specialty of forensic medicine and toxicology. Firstly, as a student and now as a teacher, I realized that the majority of the medical students find toxicology uninteresting, and many of them have a fear of the subject which they feel is difficult to remember and score. As a teacher, I make sure that my students develop a keen interest in the all-important subject of toxicology, and now this is my sincere attempt to do the same for a much larger number of medical students through this book entitled *Rapid Review of Toxicology*.

The book includes the entire toxicology syllabus as prescribed by the Medical Council of India for the 2nd year MBBS students during their learning of forensic medicine and toxicology, and also the latest topics of interest to the postgraduate medical students. The entire text is presented in a question-and-answer format with descriptions in bullets points, supplemented with good numbers of tables and flowcharts for easy understanding and memorization. The book is flooded with easy-to-remember mnemonics, and summary of important points for easy recall and quick revision. In addition, commonly asked questions in theory and practical examinations, and viva voce are included along with spotters for easy scoring in examinations.

The book is primarily meant for the undergraduates and postgraduate students of forensic medicine and toxicology, and those preparing for NEET and other postgraduate entrance examinations. Emphasis is given to the medicolegal aspects and circumstances of poisoning that will be of special interest to the forensic practitioners. Besides, it can be a useful reference source for clinicians and those dealing with toxicological emergencies.

The information presented in the text is up to date and verified from various textbooks, encyclopedias and journal articles. I hope that the students, teachers and medical practitioners find the book useful and bless this endeavor.

I am very grateful to the whole team of M/s Jaypee Brothers Medical Publishers (P) Ltd, who helped and guided me, Shri Jitendar P Vij (Group Chairman), Mr Ankit Vij (Group President), Ms Ritu Sharma (Director-Content Strategy), Ms Sunita Katla (PA to Group Chairman and Publishing Manager), Mr Manish Pahuja (General Manager-Production), Ms Samina Khan (Executive Assistant Director-Content Strategy), Mr Rajesh Sharma (Production Coordinator), Ms Seema Dogra (Cover Visualizer), Mr Rajkumar (DTP Operator), Mr Prasun Kumar (Proofreader), Mr Sumit Kumar (Team Leader-Graphic Designers) and their team members, for all their support to work in this project and make it a success. Without their cooperation, I could not have completed this project.

Constructive criticism, suggestions and contributions are welcome, and the readers can write to me at toxictanuj@gmail.com

Tanuj Kanchan

Contents

CHAPTER 1

Introduction

What is toxicology and toxinology?

Toxicology

"Toxicology" is derived from the word "toxikos" that means "poisonous". Toxicology can thus be defined as the science or study of poisons. For a more descriptive definition, toxicology refers to "*the study of properties, actions, toxicity, detection and management of poisons*".

Toxinology

Toxinology is the science or study of toxins. Toxin can be of animal, plant, or microbial origin. Toxinology thus deals with "*microbial, plant and animal toxins, and venoms*".

Differentiate between poison, toxin and venom?

Poison

Poison refers to any harmful substance which causes ill effects or death by its local and/or systemic actions. Any substance (even medicinal agents or water) can be poison. It is the dose and the intent of administration that differentiates a drug from poison.

"*Everything is poison, there is poison in everything. Only the dose makes a thing not a poison*".

-Paracelsus (The father of toxicology)

Note: Mathieu Orfila is considered as the father of modern toxicology.

Toxin

Toxins are poisons produced by some plants, animals and microorganisms that are highly toxic to other living organisms, e.g. botulinum toxin (bacterial toxin), aflatoxins (fungal toxins), saxitoxins, ciguatoxins (marine toxin), abrin, ricin, curare (phytotoxins) and venoms, etc.

Venom

Venoms are toxins of animal origin which are injected by sting, bite or body appendages. The mode of delivery of venoms is injection into the body, e.g. toxins released by venomous snakes, fishes, bees, wasps and scorpion, etc. Venoms are not toxic when ingested.

All venoms are toxins and all toxins are poisons, but all poisons are not toxins and all toxins are not venoms (Fig. 1).

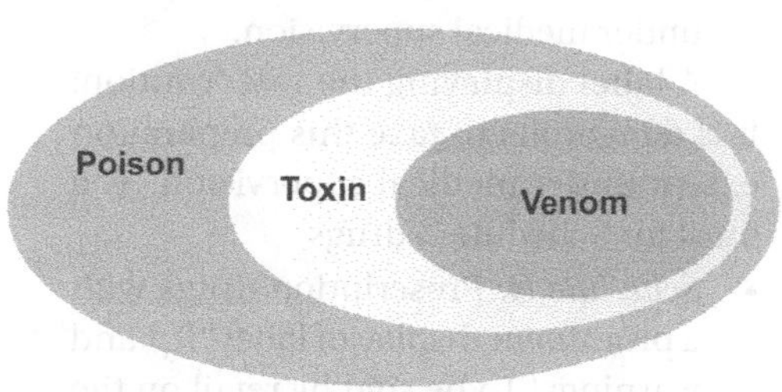

Fig. 1: Relationship between poison, toxin and venom

CHAPTER 2

Statutes in Relation to Drugs and Poisons in India

Enumerate the various acts in relation to drugs and poisons in India?

Indian Laws on drugs and poisons include:

- The Poisons Act, 1919
- The Drugs and Cosmetics Act, 1940
- The Drugs and Cosmetic Rules, 1945
- The Pharmacy Act, 1948
- The Drugs Control Act, 1950
- The Drugs and Magic Remedies Act, 1954
- The Narcotic Drugs and Psychotropic Substances (NDPS) Act, 1985
- The Prevention of Illicit Traffic in Narcotic Drugs and Psychotropic Substances Act, 1988.

Enumerate some important schedules in the Drugs and Cosmetic Rules, 1945.

The Drugs and Cosmetic Rules contain schedules listed from A to Y. Few important schedules in relation to practice of medicine are:

- *Schedule C:* Biological products such as serums.
- *Schedule E:* List of poisonous substances in alternate systems of medicine.
- *Schedule F:* List of vaccines (Part I), antisera (Part II) and diagnostic antigens (Part III).
- *Schedule G:* Drugs that must be taken under medical supervision.

  A label displaying the text "caution: It is dangerous to take this preparation except under medical supervision" is a must for Schedule G drugs.
- *Schedule H:* Prescription drugs with a prominent display of label "R_x" and warning; "To be sold by retail on the prescription of a registered medical practitioner only" (Fig. 1)

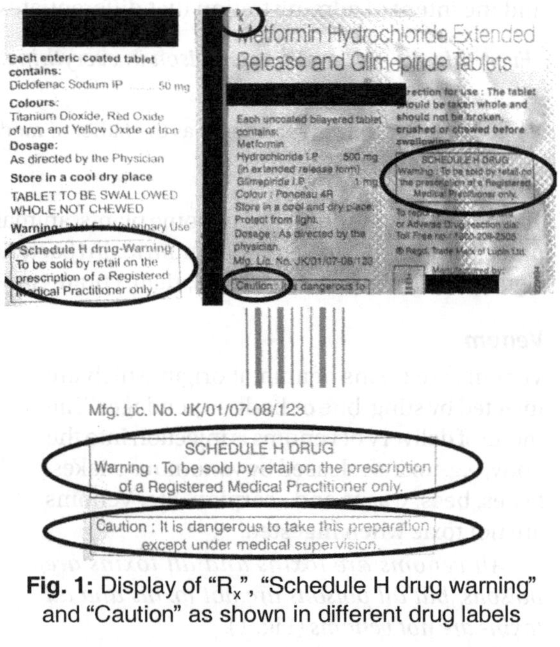

Fig. 1: Display of "R_x", "Schedule H drug warning" and "Caution" as shown in different drug labels

- *Schedule J:* No drug shall claim to treat untreatable diseases or conditions
- *Schedule R:* Condoms and other mechanical contraceptives.

Write a note on Narcotic Drugs and Psychotropic Substances (NDPS) act, 1985?

The NDPS Act came into force in order to make stricter regulations for control of the operations relating to narcotic drugs and psychotropic substances, and to implement the provisions of the International Convention on NDPS.

Narcotic drugs include *Cannabis*, coca leaf and plant, opium, poppy straw and all manufactured drugs. Psychotropic substances are included in the list specified in the schedule. The schedule lists 77 psychotropic substances and includes *lysergic acid diethylamide* (LSD), phencyclidine (PCP), amphetamines, benzodiazepines and barbiturates, etc.

The Act prohibits any person from cultivating coca, poppy or *Cannabis* plant, or producing, manufacturing, possessing, selling, purchasing, transporting, warehousing, using, consuming, or import or export of any narcotic drug or psychotropic substance, except for medical or scientific purposes and in the manner and to the extent provided by the provisions of NDPS Act or the rules or orders made thereunder.

*Prevention of illicit traffic in Narcotic Drugs and Psychotropic Substance Act, 1988 came into force to further prevent illicit traffic in NDPS.

Offences and penalties

Any violation of the provisions of the NDPS Act would attract penalties in terms of imprisonment and fine. The penalties are based on the quantity of narcotic drugs and psychotropic substances involved (Flowchart 1).

Small quantity and commercial quantity of some of the narcotic drugs and psychotropic substances are given in Table 1.

Table 1: Quantity of narcotic drugs and psychotropic substances

Agent	*Small quantity*	*Commercial quantity*
Cannabis and its resin (charas, hashish)	100 g	1 kg
Ganja	1 kg	20 kg
Coca leaf	100 g	2 kg
Cocaine	2 g	100 g
Opium	25 g	2.5 kg
Heroin or morphine	5 g	250 g
Phencyclidine (PCP)	2 g	50 g
Lysergic acid diethylamide (LSD)	0.002 g	0.1 g

Flowchart 1: Offences and penalties for contravention of the provisions of the Narcotic Drugs and Psychotropic Substances (NDPS) Act

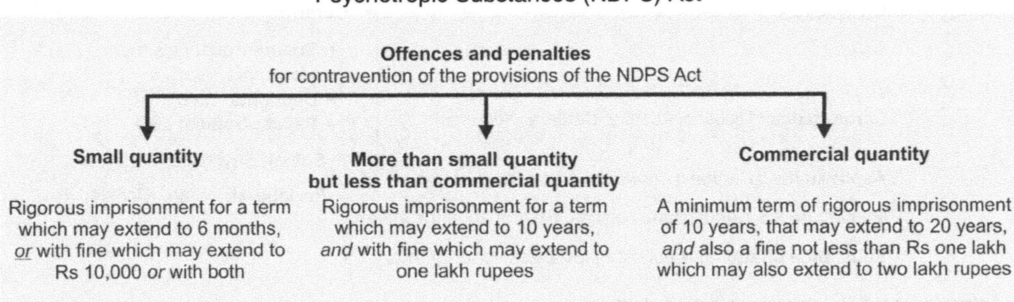

CHAPTER 3

General Principles of Toxicology

Give a detailed classification of poisons?

Poisons are often classified based on their action and principle manifestations as the following (Flowchart 1):

- **C**orrosives
- **I**rritants
- **N**eurotoxics
- **C**ardiotoxics
- **A**sphyxiants
- **M**iscellaneous
- **S**ubstance of abuse.

The **mnemonic** for remembering the classification of poisons is ***CINCAMS***.

Flowchart 1: Detailed classification of poisons

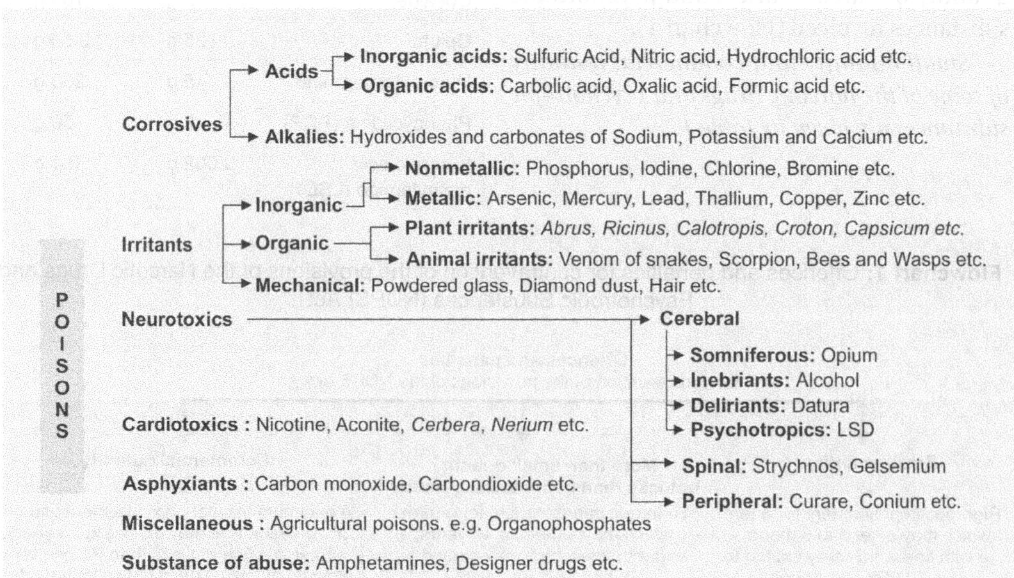

Abbreviation: LSD, Lysergic acid diethylamide

What are the various circumstances of poisoning?

Poisoning can be unintentional or intentional. Unintentional poisoning refers to accidental exposure to poisonous agents (accidental poisoning). Intentional poisoning on the other hand refers to the deliberate use of poisons for self-harm (suicidal poisoning), to harm others (homicidal poisoning), or use of poisons for other specific purposes such as to procure abortion (abortifacients), stupefy or kill the cattle or wild animals (cattle and arrow poisons), etc.

Accidental exposure to any poison is always a possibility. For example consumption of phenol or kerosene by children, consumption of poisonous fruits or plants, animal bites, etc. Similarly, any agent can be used to cause self-harm and to harm others.

Poisoning is one of the main methods of suicide in India. Agrochemicals are the most common cause of poisoning in India; aluminium phosphide and organophosphates being the commonly misused agents in North and South India respectively. Poisoning as a method of homicide is rarely reported.

Poisons can be classified based on the circumstances or motive of their use as listed here. Some of the poisonous substances in relation to the described circumstances are:

- *Homicidal poisons:* Thallium, arsenic, aconite, *Cerbera*
- *Suicidal poisons:* Organophosphates, barbiturates, rat poison
- *Abortifacients: **C**alotropis, **O**leander,* **A**conite, **L**ead (**mnemonic: *COAL***)
- *Stupefying agents: **A**tropa **b**elladonna, **C**annabis, **D**atura* (**mnemonic: *ABCD***)
- *Cattle poisons: Abrus, oleander,* strychnine, aconite, *Calotropis*
- *Arrow poisons: Abrus,* curare, strychnine, aconite, *Calotropis.*

Describe the characteristics of an ideal homicidal and an ideal suicidal poison?

Homicidal poisons should preferably be:

- Colorless, odorless, tasteless and easily mixable in food or drink (easy to administer without raising any doubt)
- Highly toxic (to ensure quick effects)
- Difficult to treat (no specific treatment or antidote to ensure the desired effect)
- Sign and symptoms should resemble a natural disease (to escape suspicion)
- Quickly destroyable, undetectable on autopsy or chemical analysis (no evidence left)
- For example thallium, arsenic, aconite, *Cerbera odollam.*

Suicidal poisons should preferably be:

- Easily available (suicide often is an impulsive act)
- Inexpensive (within the purchasing capacity of the suicide)
- Tasteless or pleasant taste, easily mixable in food or drinks (easy to consume desired amounts)
- Highly toxic (to ensure death)
- Produces quick and painless death (to ensure minimal suffering)
- For example organophosphorus compounds (OPC), aluminum phosphide, rat poison, barbiturates, etc.

Describe the possible routes of exposure and action of poison?

The 5 common routes of exposure to poisonous agents can be remembered by the **mnemonic:** ***IIIII (5 Is)***:

- Ingestion or oral (most common)
- Injection or parenteral [intramuscular (IM)/intravenous (IV)/subcutaneous (SC)/intradermal]
- Inhalation
- Introduction (per vaginal or rectal)
- Inunction (local dermal application).

Action of poisons

Action of poisons can be local or/and systemic (remote):

- *Local*: For example corrosives act locally to cause chemical destruction, mechanical irritants damage the gastrointestinal (GI) mucosa by direct action
- *Systemic*: For example action of strychnine on spinal cord, opiates on central nervous system (CNS) and digitalis on heart
- *Both local and systemic:* For example carbolic acid, oxalic acid and phosphorus, etc. have local as well as remote systemic actions.

Describe the fate and effect of poisons in a human body?

The fate of poisons in the body is shown in the Flowchart 2.

Fate of poison in body (metabolism and excretion)

- The ingested poison is absorbed, following which it is metabolized in liver and excreted mostly by kidneys. A part of the absorbed poison may be exhaled in breath or excreted through bile, sweat, saliva, tear and milk, etc.
- Some part of the poison may be removed from the body unabsorbed in vomiting or by defecation.

Poisons such as chloroform, phosphorus, nitrates and acetic acid, etc. however, are completely oxidized/evaporated/destroyed in the body and escape detection postmortem.

Flowchart 2: Route of exposure and effect of poisons in a human body

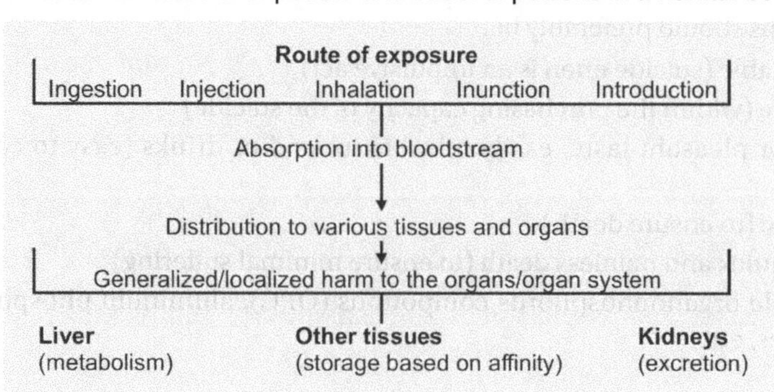

Cumulative poisons

Some poisons get accumulated in certain organs or tissues, and are retained in the body for longer periods. These poisons are known as cumulative poisons. These have an affinity to particular tissues or organs such as skin, hair, nails and bones, e.g. arsenic, mercury, lead and fluoride, etc.

Different poisons thus, can be detected in various body tissues and body fluids during postmortem for variable periods of time.

Note: Some drugs such as morphine, barbiturates, etc. after parenteral administration are resecreted in stomach. In such cases, stomach wash may be considered useful.

Describe the fate of poisons after death and their effect on putrefaction?

Some poisons modify putrefaction, while some others are modified by putrefaction.

Poisons that modify or effect putrefaction include:

Poisons which ↑ rate of putrefaction	*Poisons which ↓ rate of putrefaction*
Chronic alcoholism Hydrogen sulfide Strychnine (death after multiple seizures)	Chronic heavy metal poisoning Carbolic acid Strychnine (death after a few seizures)

Poisons that are modified or effected by putrefaction include:

Destroyed by putrefaction	*Resist putrefaction*	*Produced during putrefaction*
Aconitine Morphine	Barbiturates Corrosives, Cyanide Datura Heavy metals Nicotine Phosphorus or Organophosphates	Alcohol Carbon monoxide Cyanide

Describe the factors modifying action of poisons?

Factors modifying action of poisons

Endogenous factors (Human related)	*Exogenous factors (Poison related)*
1. Age (extremes of ages are more vulnerable) 2. Health (better tolerated by healthy persons)	1. Quantity (↑ quantity, ↑ toxicity) 2. Physical form (toxicity: gases> liquids> solids; for solids toxicity depends on solubility)
3. Stomach (↑ absorption in empty stomach) 4. Achlorhydria (No or limited HCl in gastric secretions may cause reduced toxic effects; for example cyanide salts are not converted to toxic HCN)	3. Solubility (↑ solubility, ↑ toxicity) 4. Concentration (↑ concentration, ↑ toxicity)
5. Tolerance (With continuous use, occurs ↑ tolerance and ↓ response to otherwise toxic doses; for example chronic alcoholism)	5. Route of exposure (toxicity: IV injection > inhalation > IM injection > ingestion)
6. Idiosyncrasy (individual's hypersensitivity to certain substances; toxicity may occur at non-toxic doses) 7. Coma or sleep (↓ gastric motility, ↑ absorption from stomach)	6. Nature (cumulative poisons may cause) delayed action on reaching toxic levels 7. Chemical combination (some poisons may turn to be harmless when taken together)

Note: Exceptions to the earlier described effects are:

- Ingestion of large quantities of poisons such as copper sulfate may cause excessive vomiting resulting in its elimination and thus, the amount ingested is unrelated to the toxicity
- In cases of gastrectomy, poisons reach intestine earlier and thus, the effects of poisons that are predominantly absorbed through intestine (e.g. alcohol, morphine, etc.) is faster.

Describe the types of poisoning based on the dose and duration of exposure of poison?

Based on the dose and duration of exposure, a case of poisoning may present as:

- *Fulminant poisoning:* Occurs due to intake of a massive dose. Death is very rapid
- *Acute poisoning:* Occurs due to a single large dose or multiple smaller doses in a short interval
- *Chronic poisoning:* Results from smaller doses over a long period of time
- *Subacute or subchronic poisoning:* Duration of exposure varies between that of acute and chronic poisoning and likewise the features are a mixture of acute and chronic poisoning. Types of poisoning based on the duration of exposure of poison are shown in Table 1.

Table 1: Types of poisoning based on the duration of exposure of poison

Category	Duration of exposure
Acute	<24 hours
Subacute	≤1 month
Chronic	>3 months
Subchronic	1–3 months

Describe the general diagnostic considerations in a suspected case of poisoning?

Diagnostic considerations in a suspected case of poisoning

The diagnostic considerations in a suspected case of poisoning are listed as follows:

- *History* of intake of any poisonous substance or plant, or animal or insect bite
- *Symptoms* of sudden onset such as nausea, vomiting, diarrhea, drowsiness, convulsions, delirium, unconsciousness, coma, etc. typically after consumption of food or drinks or a bite
- *Odor:* Ingestion of certain poisons produce a typical odor in breath diagnostic of that poison
- *State of pupils:* Pupils may typically be constricted or dilated in certain poisonings
- *Color of urine:* may be typical in certain poisonings. Example: Red (in mercury and lead poisoning, porphyria), brown (in nitric acid poisoning, acute tubular necrosis), olive green (in carbolic acid poisoning) and blue (in methylene blue intake)
- *Investigations:* Chemical analysis of the stomach wash, blood and urine for presence of poison remains a confirmatory criterion in diagnosis of poisoning.

Diagnosis of poisoning in the living is primarily based on the identification of toxidromes.

Specific signs and symptoms are grouped as "toxidromes" for effective management of poisoning cases. Common toxidromes described in literature are:

- *Anticholinergic*: Atropine, antidepressants, antipsychotics, antihistamines
- *Cholinergic:* Organophosphates, carbamates, nicotine, mushrooms
- *Sympathomimetic:* Amphetamine, cocaine, phencyclidine
- *Central nervous system depressants:* Alcohol, opioids, barbiturates, benzodiazepines.

Diagnosis of poisoning in the dead is based on specific autopsy observations. (color of postmortem lividity as shown in Table 2, characteristic odor of stomach contents, etc.), and chemical analysis of the viscera and body fluids for presence or absence of poisons.

Table 2: Characteristic postmortem lividity in certain poisonings

Postmortem lividity	Poisoning
Grey brown	Aniline, Nitrites, Nitrates
Cherry red or light red	Carbon monoxide
Brick pink or brick red	Cyanide
Dark or black	Opium
Brown	Phosphorus

Describe the diagnostic utility of pupillary changes and odor giving suitable examples?

Condition of pupils may help in identification of poisons. Some common examples are listed in Table 3.

Hippus (derived from Greek word referring to a horse for its rhythmic galloping movements): Hippus or spasmodic pupil denotes rhythmic intermittent dilatation and constriction of the pupils that is independent of external stimuli. This alternate constriction and dilation is observed in aconite poisoning, myasthenia gravis, multiple sclerosis and neurosyphilis, etc.

Table 3: Diagnostic utility of pupillary changes

Mydriasis (Dilated pupils)	*Miosis (Constricted pupils)*
• **A**lcohol, **A**mphetamines • ***B**elladonna* (atropine) • **C**orrosives (except phenol), **C**arbon monoxide • **D**eliriants (*Datura, Cannabis*, cocaine)	• **O**rganophosphorus compounds (**OPC**) • **O**pium (morphine) • **P**henol • **C**oma (alcoholic), **C**affeine, **C**arbamates
Mnemonic: *ABCD*	**Mnemonic: *OPC-OPC***

Pontine hemorrhage: Characterized by coma, **p**inpoint pupil, **p**yrexia and **p**oor prognosis. **Mnemonic: *3Ps***

Macewen's sign

The pupils are constricted in coma due to alcohol intoxication. External stimulus such as pinching the skin of face or neck causes transient dilation of the pupils. The sign though suggested to be useful in differentiating coma resulting from alcohol intoxication versus that of head injury is obsolete and rarely used in clinical practice.

Some poisons impart characteristic odor in breath or gastric contents that may help in identification of the poisons (Table 4).

Table 4: Poisons that impart characteristic odor

Odor	*Poison*
Bitter almond	Cyanide, hydrogen cyanide, nitrobenzene
Burnt rope	*Cannabis*
Garlicky	**P**hosphorus, **O**rganophosphates, **T**hallium, **A**rsenic (**Mnemonic *POTA***)
Fishy	Zinc and aluminum phosphide
Rotten egg	Hydrogen sulfide
Fruity	Alcohol, solvents
Sweet	Chloroform (halogenated hydrocarbons)
Kerosene like	Kerosene, organophosphates or carbamates (solvents)
Phenolic	Carbolic acid, lysol, etc.

Describe the general principles in management of a case of poisoning? Write a note on Scandinavian method of treatment of poisoning?

General principles in management of poisoning:

- Exposure reduction (removal from the source of exposure and wash the exposed parts)
- Assessment of patient's condition
- ABCD management (**a**irway, **b**reathing, **c**irculation, **d**epression of CNS)
- Decontamination (elimination of poison)

- Administering antidotes (specific treatment)
- Symptomatic treatment
- Reassurance and general nursing care
- Counseling.

Scandinavian method of treatment of poisoning

A method based on intensive supportive theory that is known to decrease mortality substantially.

- *Assessment of patient:* Staging of unconsciousness (CNS), assessment of shock (CVS), breathing (RS) and body temperature
- *Emergency measures:* Management of cardiorespiratory failure, and preventing further absorption of poison
- *General care:* For control of hypothermia, fluid electrolyte imbalance, infections and general nursing care.

Write a note on role of symptomatic treatment in management of poisoning?

In most cases of suspected poisonings, the emergency physicians are unaware about the poison consumed. Even when poison is known or identified, specific antidotes are not available for more than 90% of the poisons.

The basic approach is to treat the patient and not the poison (not all poisons have antidotes).

The management of poisoning is mostly symptomatic. A few commonly observed symptoms and their treatment are listed here:

Symptoms	*Treatment*
Coma or Central nervous system depression	Coma cocktail*
Respiratory failure	Oxygen therapy
Circulatory failure	Dopamine
Hypovolemia	Plenty of fluids
Metabolic acidosis	Sodium bicarbonate
Convulsions	Diazepam or short-acting barbiturates
Anxiety	Anxiolytics
Pyrexia	Antipyretics

Coma cocktail: Hoffman and Goldfrank suggested IV administration of **naloxone** (2 mg), **dextrose** solution and **thiamine** (100 mg) for effective management of comatose patients in cases of unknown poisoning.

Mnemonic for constituents of coma cocktail: ***NDT or Do Not Trouble***

Besides, treat hypothermia or hyperthermia and fluid and electrolyte imbalances appropriately.

Describe in brief the general measures of decontamination?

Decontamination is done to promote elimination or excretion of poison and ensure that the absorption of the poison is reduced. Process of decontamination may vary based on the route of exposure and part of the body involved. Common methods of decontamination are:

- **For unabsorbed poisons (by elimination):**
  - *Inhaled poisons (inhalational decontamination):* Remove from the source of exposure and ensure adequate ventilation. Artificial respiration and oxygen therapy may follow if required.

- *Contact poison (ocular or dermal decontamination):* Wash the affected part with water and neutralize the poison with specific chemical.
- *Ingested poison (gut or gastrointestinal decontamination):* Gastrointestinal decontamination comprises of gastric lavage, emesis, whole bowel irrigation, administration of single-dose or multidose activated charcoal, cathartics, etc.

- **For absorbed poisons (by excretion):**
  - *Diuresis (forced):* Increase urination by giving lot of water (when renal functions are normal).
  - *Diaphoresis:* Increase perspiration or sweating when renal functions are compromised (no longer used).
  - *Dialysis:* Peritoneal as well as hemodialysis.
  - Charcoal hemoperfusion
  - Chelating agents (described on page 16 as specific treatment for heavy metal poisoning).

Note: Hemodialysis is useful in poisoning with **l**ithium, **a**lcohol (ethyl and methyl), **s**alicylates, **t**heophylline, **b**arbiturates, etc.

Mnemonic for poisons requiring hemodialysis: ***LAST Barbiturates or LAST Barb or BLAST.***

Describe the various methods of gastrointestinal decontamination (GID) Or Write a note on gastric lavage (GL), emesis, whole bowel irrigation (WBI) and administration of activated charcoal (AC)?

Gastric lavage or stomach wash

Gastric lavage tube (Fig. 1)

- *Adults:* Ewald tube/Boas tube/Jacques tube. 1.5 meter long and 0.5 inches in diameter. (Levin tube used in carbolic acid poisoning)
- *Children:* Orogastric tube or Ryle's tube.

Note: Lavacuator tubes have replaced older tubes, and are used in emergency rooms for lavage.

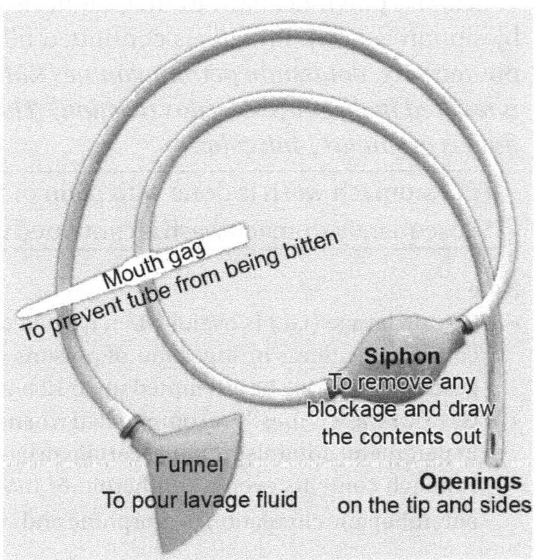

Fig. 1: Gastric lavage tube

Gastric lavage

- *Indication:* Ingested poisons.
- *Preferred time:* Within 2–4 hours of ingestion.
- *Preferred route:* Oral (nasal insertion can cause nasal mucosa damage).
- *Preferred position of the patient:* Left lateral (foot end elevated to minimize the chances of aspiration).
- *Length of tube to be inserted:*
  - *Adults:* 50 cms
  - *Children:* 25 cms

Procedure

Patient lies in left lateral position with foot end elevated

↓

Inserting end of the tube is well lubricated and passed through mouth into the stomach.

↓

Ensure cooperation from a conscious patient. Ideally the patient should be sedated and intubated before the procedure. In unconscious patients, procedure is carried out after endotracheal intubation to ensure protection of airways and prevent aspiration.

↓

Ensure that the tube has reached stomach and not airways

- If the tube reaches the airways, it may cause cough in conscious patients
- Free end of the tube is put in a water container; bubbles are released if tube is in airways
- Confirmation by air insufflation and auscultation over epigastric area for peculiar sounds
- Small amount of stomach contents may be aspirated for pH testing to confirm the location.

↓

Tepid water (38°C) is poured through funnel (approximately 300 mL in adults or approximately 100 mL in children at a time)

↓

Tube is pinched below funnel; funnel is lowered and pressure released (the fluid drains out by siphon action). Process is continued till the returning fluid becomes clear (alike the fluid poured), *e.g. potassium permanganate ($KMnO_4$) loses its pink color as it oxidizes the poison and is reduced in the process (redox reaction). The stomach wash hence, is continued till the returning fluid is of similar pink color.*

First stomach wash is done with plain or tap water and preserved for chemical analysis. Subsequently stomach wash is continued with saline or any specific lavage fluid as indicated.

Note

- Gastric lavage (GL) is useful when carried out within 2–4 hours of ingestion of poisons. In cases of comatose patients or ingestion of poisons that reduce gastric motility (salicylates and morphine) gastric lavage may be attempted up to 12 hours after ingestion of poison.
- Gastric lavage is mostly recommended when the poison is taken orally. However, GL may also be useful in parenteral administration of certain drugs or poison. For example morphine that may be found in stomach contents even when heroin or morphine is administered parenteral. This is attributed to enterohepatic circulation of morphine and subsequent reflux of duodenal contents into the stomach.

Lavage fluids (commonly used)

- Tepid or lukewarm water
- Saline (0.9%)
- Oxidizing agents such as $KMnO_4$ (1:5000 dilution) and 4% tannic acid.

Lavage fluids recommended in specific poisonings

- *Castor oil and warm water:* Carbolic acid poisoning
- *Calcium gluconate or lime water:* Oxalic acid poisoning

- *25% sodium thiosulfate solution:* Cyanide poisoning
- *1% potassium ferrocyanide:* Copper poisoning (forms insoluble cupric ferrocyanide).

Complications of gastric lavage
- Vomiting
- Vagal inhibition
- Esophageal or gastric mucosal injury
- Aspiration pneumonia
- Cardiac arrhythmias
- Perforation
- Convulsions
- Laryngospasm
- Water intoxication.

Contraindications for gastric large
Absolute contraindication (lavage is not to be tried at all):
- Corrosives (GL in inorganic acid poisonings can result in perforation of already fragile gastric mucosa leading to fatal peritonitis)

Note: Exception is carbolic acid poisoning where the mucosa is thick and leathery and lavage can be done.

Relative contraindication (lavage to be tried only after prior precautions to protect from the associated risks):
- **C**omatose (risk of aspiration)
- **H**emorrhagic diathesis (risk of bleeding)
- **E**sophageal varices (risk of bleeding)
- **C**onvulsions (risk of aspiration)
- **K**erosene and other volatile poisons (risk of aspiration)
- **C**hildren (risk of injury with Ewald tube)
- **C**ardiac arrhythmias (risk of sudden death).

To minimize the possible risks, patient should be sedated and intubated before lavage is tried.

Mnemonic: *Contraindications of gastric lavage*

Absolute: *C except C (Corrosives except carbolic acid)*

Relative: *CHECK CC (as elaborated above)*

Emesis (induction of vomiting)

Vomiting can only be induced in conscious patients when medullary centers are responsive, and when no other facilities are available. Care should be taken to prevent aspiration of gastric contents. *Emesis is no longer practiced in management of poisoning.*

Methods used to induce vomiting
- By tickling the back of the throat with finger, spoon, etc. (considered as a safe method)
- Use of household emetics
  - Consuming large amount of warm water or saline
  - Freshly prepared solution of black mustard powder in water.

- Ipecacuanha powder or ipecac syrup (drug of choice to induce vomiting)
  - *Source:* Root of *Cephaelis ipecacuanha*
  - *Active principle:* Cephaeline, emetine
  - *Dose:* Adults: 30 mL, children: 10–15 mL with water.

Contraindications
- *Absolute:* Coma, convulsions, corrosives, kerosene and volatile poisons
- *Relative:* Infants, advanced pregnancy, severe heart diseases and foreign body ingestion.

Whole bowel irrigation (WBI)

Purpose
To hasten the passage of ingested poisons through the GI tract and cleanse the bowel.

Irrigation fluid
Large volumes of polyethylene glycol-electrolyte solution (PEG-ES).

Route
Orally or using a nasogastric tube.

Indications
- In body packers for the passage of drug packets
- Iron or lithium ingestion in large quantities
- Ingestion of sustained-release or enteric-coated drugs in large quantities
- Delayed presentation to the hospital (>2 hours) after ingestion of poison.

Contraindications
- Bowel obstruction, perforation, ileus, GI hemorrhage, hemodynamic instability, uncontrolled vomiting, coma and compromised airway reflexes
- Infants, elderly, or debilitated patients may not tolerate the WBI procedure well.

Activated charcoal: use of single-dose or multidose activated charcoal

Activated charcoal (AC) is obtained by destructive distillation of carbonaceous substance such as wood followed by steam activation or heating with an activating agent such as steam, carbon dioxide, etc.

Purpose
Adsorption of poison on its surface, that minimizes the absorption of poison in the GIT.

Dosage
1 g/kg body weight (25–100 g in adults) as a single dose.

Procedure
Activated charcoal is mixed with water to form a slurry or suspension and administered orally or through orogastric or nasogastric tube.

Indications
In poisons that are adsorbed; preferably within 1–2 hours of ingestion.

Contraindications

Bowel obstruction, ileus, coma, convulsions, compromised airway reflexes, corrosives, kerosene, and volatile poisons.

Complications

Aspiration is the most serious complication.

Note: Administration of AC is not useful in poisoning with alcohols, corrosives, kerosene, iron and lithium, etc. as these are poorly adsorbed on AC.

Multidose activated charcoal (MDAC)

When two or more doses of activated charcoal are administered.

Indications

Poisonings involving:

- Sustained-release preparations
- Drugs with enterohepatic or enteroenteric circulation
- Decreased gastric motility or increased GI transit time.

Write a note on antidotes, its types and their role in management of poisoning?

Antidotes are substances which neutralize or counteract the effect of poisons.

Antidotes can be classified into three groups based on their primary mechanism of action:

1. *Mechanical or physical antidotes:* Neutralize poisons by mechanical action and prevent their absorption.
   a. *Activated charcoal:* Adsorbs and retains the poison thus, delaying their absorption
   b. *Demulcents:* E.g. milk, oil, egg white, etc. from a protective covering over gastric mucosa thus preventing it from toxic effects of poisons and also delay their absorption.

   Note: Demulcents should not be given in poisons with affinity to fat such as phosphorus, phenol, organophosphates, kerosene, dichlorodiphenyltrichloroethane (DDT), etc.

   c. *Bulky foods* such as boiled rice, mashed bananas and vegetables, etc. are useful in cases of ingestion of mechanical irritants such as powdered glass and diamond dust, etc. Bulky foods engulf the mechanical irritants thus, protecting mucosa from any possible injury and facilitates its excretion.
2. *Chemical antidotes:* Act chemically with poisons to form nontoxic complexes.
   a. Alkali neutralizes acid and vice versa (weak acids and alkalis are used)
   b. Potassium permanganate (1:5000 solution) is used as an oxidizing agent in poisoning of phosphorous, opium, strychnine, etc.
   c. Tannic acid (4% solution) is useful in poisoning of strychnine, nicotine, cocaine, aconite and metallic poisons such as lead, mercury, copper, zinc, etc.
   d. Lugol's iodine or tincture iodine solution used in poisoning of lead, mercury, strychnine, etc.
   e. Copper sulfate in phosphorus poisoning; precipitates it as harmless copper phosphide
   f. Calcium compounds are used to precipitate oxalates in oxalic acid poisoning.

3. *Physiological or pharmacological antidotes:* Produces effect that is opposite to those produced by the poison or reverses the effects of poison by acting in a certain manner.
   a. Physostigmine is an ideal physiological antidote for atropine poisoning.
   b. Amyl nitrite is the physiological antidote for cyanide poisoning.
   c. Barbiturates are physiological antidote for strychnine poisoning.

   Some of the common poisons, their antidotes and mechanism of action are listed here:

Poisoning	*Antidotes*	*Mechanism of action*
Cyanides	Thiosulfate	Accelerated detoxification
Paracetamol	Acetylcysteine	Accelerated detoxification
Methanol	Ethanol, fomepizole	Reduced toxic conversion
Ethylene glycol	Ethanol, fomepizole	Reduced toxic conversion
Morphine or opium	Naloxone	Receptor site competition
Organophosphates	Atropine	Receptor site blockade
Carbon monoxide	Oxygen	Toxic effect bypass
Cyanide	Oxygen	Toxic effect bypass
Thallium	Prussian blue	Inert complex formation
Copper	Penicillamine	Inert complex formation
Heavy meals (in general)	Chelating agents	Inert complex formation

Note: Antidotes such as atropine (for organophosphate poisoning), ethanol (for methanol poisoning), copper sulfate (for phosphorus poisoning), barbiturates (for strychnine poisoning), and chelating agents (for heavy metal poisoning), etc. are potentially toxic and hence, should be administered judiciously.

Write a note on universal antidote?

Universal antidote refers to a combination of mechanical and chemical antidotes that can be administered when the exact nature of poison is unknown.

It constitutes of a mixture of two parts activated charcoal, one part tannic acid, and one part magnesium oxide.

Household alternative includes a mixture of burnt toast, liquid tea and milk of magnesia.

Constituents	*Household alternative*	*Composition*	*Purpose (for)*
Activated charcoal	Burnt toast	2 parts (50%)	Adsorbs poisons
Tannic acid	Strong liquid tea	1 part (25%)	Oxidize poisons
Magnesium oxide	Milk of magnesia	1 part (25%)	Neutralizes acid

Mnemonic (universal antidote): *ATM in the ratio 2:1:1*

Universal antidote is an outdated concept and is no longer recommended.

At times, people refer to activated charcoal (AC) alone as universal antidote.

Write a note on chelating agents?

Chelating agents

These are substances which form a stable, nontoxic, soluble and cyclic complex with heavy metals rendering it inactive and facilitating its excretion. These agents are used in treatment of heavy metal poisoning. Some of the commonly used chelating agents are:

- *BAL (British anti-lewisite, dimercaprol):*
  - Effective in poisoning with arsenic, mercury, lead (along with EDTA).

- British anti-lewisite (BAL) in oil is given by *deep IM injection only*
- British anti-lewisite is hepatotoxic; so contraindicated in hepatic insufficiency.

Note: British anti-lewisite in oil contains dimercaprol, benzyl benzoate and peanut oil.

- *Ethylenediaminetetraacetic acid (EDTA), edetic acid, calcium disodium versenate, versene:*
  - Effective in lead poisoning. May be used in poisoning of mercury, copper, aluminum, etc.
  - Administered usually as *IV infusion.*
- *D-Penicillamine (cuprimine, dimethyl cysteine):*
  - Drug of choice in copper poisoning (copperiedus)
  - Also effective in lead and mercury poisoning
  - Administered *orally.*
- *Deferoxamine (desferrioxamine):*
  - Drug of choice in acute and chronic iron poisoning, and in aluminium toxicity.
  - Oral or IM administration. IV administration only in cases of shock (slow IV infusion)

Note: *Deferoxamine is secreted by bacteria Streptomyces pilosus.*

- Dimercaptosuccinic acid (DMSA)
- 2,3-Dimercapto-1-propanesulfonic acid (DMPS)

DMSA and DMPS are newer and safer chelating agents preferred in treatment of acute lead, arsenic and mercury poisoning.

Write a note on sampling and preservation of body fluids and viscera in a suspected case of poisoning? Mention the limitations of preservatives commonly used for preservation of viscera or biological tissues at autopsy?

The choice and collection of body fluids and viscera at autopsy for toxicological analysis is based on the route and fate of the poison administered. Ingestion or oral route is most commonly encountered in fatal poisonings and hence, choice of specimens collected routinely at autopsy is based on the passage or movement of the poison and its breakdown products in the body as shown in the Flowchart 3.

Flowchart 3: Sampling and preservation of body fluids and viscera in a suspected case of poisoning

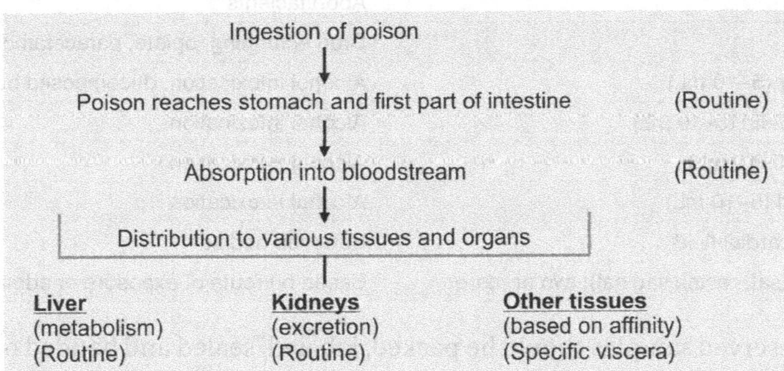

Following body tissues or fluids commonly referred to as "routine viscera" are preserved routinely in all suspected cases of poisoning by ingestion for toxicological analysis (Table 5) at the Regional Forensic Science Laboratory (RFSL).

Table 5: Management of routine viscera for toxicological analysis

Biological tissues or fluids routinely preserved	*Preservative*
Stomach with its contents Proximal 30 cm of small intestine with contents Liver with gall bladder (500 gms) Kidney (half of each kidney)	*Rectified spirit* (preservative of choice) *Saturated solution of common salt* (most commonly used for its easy availability, cost-effectiveness, and low misuse potential)
Blood (20 mL) from femoral or subclavian vein Urine (50 mL) from bladder directly	*Sodium fluoride and potassium oxalate* *Sodium fluoride or thymol*

Note: 10 mg/mL of sodium fluoride (enzyme inhibitor) along with 3 mg/mL of potassium oxalate (anticoagulant) when used to preserve blood, protects it from postmortem bacterial production of alcohols. Sodium fluoride can be used as preservative for all body fluids.

Heart blood may be acceptable sample for qualitative analysis of poisons but not the quantitative analysis as the poison/toxic concentration may be increased due to redistribution.

In addition to the "routine viscera", certain body fluids and viscera need to be preserved for toxicological analysis based on the route of exposure, affinity and type of poison. Such samples are referred as "specific viscera" (Table 6).

Table 6: Indications for specific viscera in toxicological analysis

Specific biological tissues or fluids	*Indications*
Brain (one hemisphere)	Cerebral and spinal poisons, cyanide poisoning
Spinal cord (entire length)	Spinal poisons
Lungs (whole)	Solvent abuse, inhaled or volatile poisons
Heart (whole)	Strychnine poisoning, cardiac poisons
Bone (entire long bone)	Chronic heavy metal poisoning
Hair (20–30 strands) and nails (whole)	Chronic heavy metal poisoning, drugs of abuse
Fat tissue (from abdominal wall)	Anesthetic agents, pesticide poisoning
Muscle tissue (100 gm, preferably quadriceps)	Exhumed and decomposed bodies, cocaine
Skin and subcutaneous fat ($2 \times 2 \times 1$ cm^3)	Injected poisons, snake bite, anesthetic deaths
Uterus (whole)	Abortifacients
Bile (20 mL)	Drug screening, opiate, paracetamol poisoning
Vitreous humor (5–10 mL)	Alcohol intoxication, decomposed bodies
Cerebrospinal fluid (5–10 mL)	Alcohol intoxication
Synovial fluid (5–10 mL)	Alcohol intoxication
Pericardial fluid (5–10 mL)	Alcohol intoxication
Pleural or pericardial fluid	Putrefied bodies
Swabs (intranasal, rectal, vaginal); two or more	Based on route of exposure or administration

All the preserved samples should be packed, labeled, sealed and handed over to the police personnel for toxicological analysis at the RFSL thus, maintaining the chain of custody.

Limitations of preservatives commonly used for preservation at autopsy

- Rectified spirit is not indicated in organic acid (phenol, oxalic acid, etc.) and paraldehyde poisoning as these agents are soluble in the preservative

- Rectified spirit is not indicated in suspected alcohol poisoning or intoxication as its use may result in false positive or erroneous results
- Rectified spirit interferes with the luminescence property of phosphorus, hence not recommended
- Saturated solution of common salt is not indicated in plant poisons, aconite and mineral acid poisoning.

Note: Viscera meant for toxicological analysis should never be preserved in formalin. Formalin caused fixation of tissue and hence, extraction of poison becomes difficult.

Write a short note on entomotoxicology?

Entomotoxicology

Entomotoxicology is a combined application of entomology (study of insects) and toxicology (study of nature and effects of poison) in forensic investigations. Entomotoxicology refers to the analysis of drugs and poisons in insects that feed on the dead bodies.

Forensic applications

- *To determine if a certain drug or poison was present in the body at the time of death:* With advanced putrefaction and skeletonization, extraction and analysis of drugs and poisons becomes increasingly difficult because of the lack of suitable body fluids and tissues. However, maggots feeding on a corpse can be analyzed for the presence of drugs or poison such as *cocaine, opiates and malathion,* etc. in the dead body by mass spectrometry.
- *More accurate estimation of postmortem interval:* Size of the maggots gives a clue to the postmortem interval (PMI); more the size of fly larva, more is the PMI.

Maggots feeding on corpses dying of drug overdose, however, may grow abnormally large due to the stimulant effect of drug or poison on maggots. Thus, there is a likelihood of erroneous PMI estimates based on the size of maggots alone, unless these are analyzed for presence/absence of any poisons. These large sized maggots are referred to as "super maggots" (Flowchart 4).

Note: Malathion is shown to be responsible for delayed arrival of flies thus, effecting PMI estimate.

Flowchart 4: Formation of 'Super maggots'

Death from cocaine/ drug overdose → Maggots feed on the dead body → Cocaine/drugs taken up by maggots → Cocaine/drugs increase rate of metabolism → Increased feeding → Increased size of maggots "Super maggots"

Medicolegal Duties of Doctor in an Alleged Case of Poisoning

CHAPTER 4

Describe the medicolegal duties of a doctor in an alleged case of poisoning?

Medical practitioners owe certain clinical or medical and legal responsibilities in cases of alleged poisoning as described here.

Clinical or medical duties

The primary duty of a doctor is to save the life of the patient and hence, an accurate assessment of patient's condition and prompt treatment (symptomatic as well as specific) remains the mainstay. General principles of diagnosis and management in this regard, are described in the previous chapter.

It is the duty of the doctor to collect appropriate samples such as blood, urine, and gastric washings, etc. as part of clinical investigations and for investigative purposes.

Legal duties

Medical practitioners are duty bound to act in a certain way while dealing with a case of alleged poisoning in accordance with the administrative guidelines and legal statutes. The duties of a doctor in this regard include:

- *Intimation:* Every case of poisoning admitted in the government hospitals is to be reported to the police.

  For private practitioners, it is obligatory to report all cases of homicidal poisoning. Though, they are under no legal obligation to report accidental and suicidal cases, it is advisable they do so.

  In cases of food poisoning, the public health authorities must be notified in addition to informing the police.
- *Documentation:* Detailed documentation of the history, investigations, management and other relevant information is expected, and such medicolegal records should be preserved securely.
- *Preservation:* Doctor should collect and preserve appropriate samples or evidentiary material such as blood, urine, feces, vomitus, first gastric wash, contaminated clothing, and alleged drugs or poison consumed, contaminated food, etc. for chemical analysis at the Regional Forensic Science Laboratories (RFSLs).
- *Communications with the police or investigative authorities:* The doctor is expected to divulge any information concerned with poisoning that is sought by the investigating officer. Professional secrecy cannot be an excuse for withholding information in such cases.

- *Dying declaration:* If the patient is critical following homicidal poisoning, arrangements should be made for recording of the dying declaration by the magistrate. Doctor needs to certify that the patient is in *compos mentis* to give a statement.
- *Death intimation and certification:* All deaths due to poisoning irrespective of the manner (suicide/accident/homicide) and place of admission (private or government) are to be reported to the police.
  Death certificate should not be issued in any of such cases.
- *Autopsy:* Postmortem examination should be carried out on requisition from the police and relevant samples should be preserved for chemical analysis at the RFSL as discussed in the previous chapter.

Mnemonic

The legal duties of a doctor can be remembered by any of the following mnemonics:
- In Dr Pillay's center death is declared intimated and autopsied
- Preserve intimate documents and communications about dying declarations, death intimations and autopsies.

Legal provisions in relation to dealing with poisoning cases

- In India, all poisoning cases are marked as medicolegal case (MLC)
- Doctor is legally bound to report homicidal poisoning and offences relating to adulteration of food and drugs, etc. to police or magistrate in accordance with *Section 39 Criminal Procedure Code (CrPC)*
- Failure on the part of doctor to report such cases is punishable under *Section 176 Indian Penal Code (IPC)*
- Intentional omission to give information of offence by doctor is punishable under *Section 202 IPC*
- As per *Section 175 CrPC*, the investigating officer has the power to summon the doctor and seek relevant information about any MLC, including the poisoning cases
- Causing disappearance of evidence of offence, or giving false information to screen offender is punishable under *Section 201 IPC.*

CHAPTER 5

Corrosives

Classify corrosive agents with suitable examples? Describe in general, the differentiating features following ingestion of corrosive acids and alkalis?

Corrosives cause extensive burns and tissue damage of the skin surface or mucous membrane it comes in contact with.

The word *caustic* refers to any substance which is corrosive in nature and thus, includes both corrosive acids and alkalis.

Classification of corrosive agents in given in the Flowchart 1.

Flowchart 1: Classification of corrosive agents

Corrosives

Corrosive acids	Corrosive alkalis
"Lick the esophagus and bite the stomach"	*"Bite the esophagus and lick the stomach"*
Cause coagulation necrosis	Cause liquefaction necrosis
Gastric involvement is more	Esophageal involvement is more
Esophageal involvement is less	Gastric involvement is less
Less viscous; rapidly passes through esophagus	More viscous; larger contact with esophagus
Columnar epithelium of stomach is susceptible	Squamous epithelium of esophagus is effected
Acid hematin formation	Alkali hematin formation
Lower risk of perforation (except conc. H_2SO_4)	Higher risk of perforation
Steroid therapy of limited value	Steroid therapy prevents stricture formation

Examples (corrosive acids)

Inorganic or mineral acids (local action)
- Sulfuric acid (H_2SO_4)
- Nitric acid (HNO_3)
- Hydrochloric acid (HCl)

Organic acids (local and remote action)
- Carbolic Acid or phenol (C_6H_5OH)
- Oxalic acid ($C_2H_2O_4$)
- Formic acid (HCOOH)

Examples (corrosive alkalis)
- Sodium hydroxide
- Potassium hydroxide
- Calcium hydroxide
- Ammonium hydroxide
- Sodium carbonate
- Potassium carbonate
- Ammonium carbonate

Discuss the clinical manifestations of mineral acid poisoning and its management?

Clinical manifestations

In general, the signs and symptoms following ingestion of mineral acids (H_2SO_4, HNO_3 or HCl) can be summarized and remembered as **mnemonic *SLUDGE***:

- **S**treaks (black) from mouth and angle of jaws, **S**alivation, **S**wollen lips, **S**odden tongue. In cases of **S**urvival; **S**cars, **S**trictures (gastric), and **S**tenosis
- **L**ip excoriation
- **U**lceration and corrosion of skin and gastrointestinal (GI) mucosa
- **D**ysphagia, **D**yspepsia, **D**ysphonia, **D**ilated pupils, **D**izziness
- **G**astrointestinal symptoms: Nausea, vomiting (brown-black mucoid), epigastric pain, constipation
- **E**xcoriation, **E**ructations, **E**yes sunken, dilated pupils, blindness (in direct exposure).

Acid burns mostly involve antrum and pylorus. Pyloric spasm prevents duodenal involvement (Fig. 1).

Distinct and specific features of the three inorganic or mineral acids are listed in Table 1.

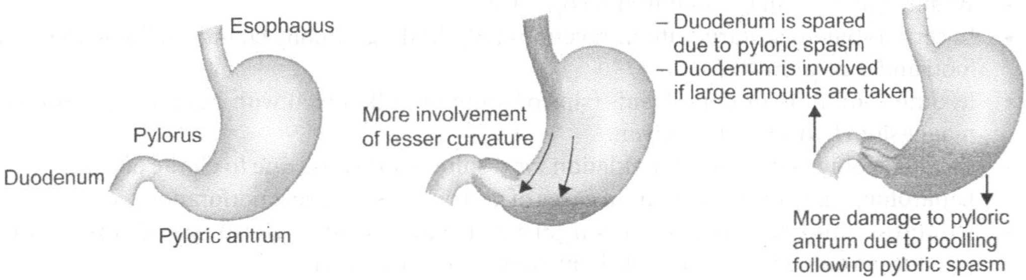

Fig. 1: Involvement of stomach and intestines in mineral acid poisoning

Table 1: Distinct and specific features of the three inorganic or mineral acids

	Conc. H_2SO_4	*Conc. HNO_3*	*Conc. HCl*
Alternative names	Oil of vitriol Battery acid	Aqua fortis Red spirit of nitre	Muriatic acid Spirit of salts
Symptoms	+++ (severe)	++ (milder)	++ (milder)
Fuming liquid	No	Yes	Yes
Abdominal distension	– –	++	++
Respiratory symptoms	– –	++	++
Tongue	Sodden black	Yellowish	Grayish
Teeth	Chalky white	Yellowish	Chalky-white
Corrosive staining	Black or dark brown	Yellowish	Grayish-white
Gastric mucosa	Wet blotting paper like	Yellowish green	Inflamed
GI perforation	Common	Less common	Uncommon
Fatal dose	5–10 mL	10–15 mL	15–20 mL
Fatal period	12–24 hours	12–24 hours	12–24 hours

Abbreviations: GI, gastrointestinal; HCl, hydrochloric acid; HNO_3, nitric acid; H_2SO_4, sulfuric acid

- Nitric acid and HCl are fuming liquids. Inhalation of fumes may cause sneezing, coughing, dyspnea, shortness of breath, tightness of chest, choking and asphyxia, cyanosis, rapid pulse, low blood pressure (BP), dizziness and weakness
- Fumes may also affect eyes resulting in lacrimation and photophobia.

Note: ***Xanthoproteic reaction:*** Nitric acid reacts with organic matter or tissue proteins and forms trinitrophenol or picric acid that causes yellowish discoloration of the skin, tongue, teeth and mucus membrane.

Management

Specific investigations

- Upper GI endoscopy to assess the mucosal damage and burns of esophagus and stomach
- Evaluation of strictures using barium swallow studies, upper GI endoscopy and computed tomography (CT) scan
- Bronchoscopy for assessment of burns in the respiratory tract in inhalation of HNO_3 or HCl.
- Chest X-ray in cases of inhalation and suspected infections.

Treatment

- Washing of the skin frequently and copiously.
- In serious patients, starts with intravenous (IV) fluids; gradually change to liquid diet, soft food and regular meals.
- In others, dilution or demulcents (sips of water or milk mixed with calcium hydroxide or magnesium hydroxide) are given.
- Tracheostomy and assisted ventilation for respiratory distress due to glottic edema.
- Laparotomy and surgical repair in cases of gastric or esophageal perforation.
- Dilatation and reconstructive surgery as treatment for strictures and obstruction (corticosteroids have limited role in prevention of strictures).
- Prednisolone and dopamine for correction of shock.
- Antibiotics (for any infection).
- Analgesics (to alleviate pain).
- Surgical debridement of burnt skin, and surgical removal of a part of the esophagus or stomach may be required.
- *Airway support:* Intubation and assisted ventilation is required in HNO_3 and HCl poisoning that causes serious inhalation injuries and pulmonary edema.

Note: In treatment of mineral acid poisoning, say NO to the following:
- No gastric lavage (as it may cause perforation of the paper thin mucosa)
- No emesis (as it may increase the risk of aspiration causing serious respiratory damage)
- No neutralization with alkalis (large amount of liberated heat may cause further damage)
- No charcoal therapy (charcoal does not adsorb caustics)
- No oral feeds where GI mucosa is severely damaged.

Cause of death

- *Immediate death* due to edema glottis and circulatory failure
- *Early death* from gastric perforation and resultant chemical peritonitis or toxemia (Death due to perforation and chemical peritonitis is uncommon in HNO_3 and HCl poisoning. Instead death can result from asphyxia due to inhalation effects of these fuming liquids)
- *Delayed death* may occur from secondary infections, pneumonia, and complications such as stricture formation.

Describe the autopsy observations and medicolegal significance in mineral acid poisoning?

Postmortem appearances

External

- Clothing is examined for stains and any damage due to burns. Yellow stains may be seen on clothing in HNO_3 poisoning
- Characteristic circumoral burns are seen in cases of ingestion. Brown black appearance of burnt and corroded skin (chin, angle of mouth, throat, hands) and mucus membrane (lips and oral mucosa) is characteristic
- Chalky-white teeth in H_2SO_4 poisoning and yellowish teeth in HNO_3 poisoning.

Internal

- Generalized corrosion and inflammation of the GI mucosa
- Ridges are more commonly involved than furrows (difference from postmortem lividity)
- Gastric mucosa has a brown or black appearance (yellow green in HNO_3 poisoning)
- Wet blotting paper consistency of gastric mucosa in H_2SO_4 poisoning
- Perforation may occur with resulting chemical peritonitis and corrosion of organs
- Corrosion and inflammation of larynx and trachea
- Pulmonary congestion and edema is characteristic of HNO_3 poisoning.

Medicolegal significance

- Most of the cases are due to suicidal ingestion
- Accidental ingestion may occur especially in children
- Homicidal use of mineral acids is rare
- Vitriolage.

Write a short note on vitriolage?

Vitriolage (vitriol throwing)

"Vitriolage" refers to intentional throwing of an acid or any corrosive agent on to the face or body of another individual with a motive to harm or disfigure or blind him or her by producing chemical burns or injuries.

The term "vitriolage" originates from "oil of vitriol" owing to the fact that concentrated H_2SO_4 is most commonly used in the act. This preference is primarily owed to its easy availability.

Epidemiology

Cases are reported worldwide; more commonly in Asian subcontinent and Jamaica.

Victim profile

Most of the victims are females and hence, often labeled as "gender crime" in Asian subcontinent. Males, however, are reported as equally common victim of vitriolage in Jamaica and other parts of the world.

Perpetrators

Mostly disgruntled lovers, or spouses in marital discord.

Motive or intent

Revenge or jealousy to harm or disfigure a person.

Predisposing factors

Rejected romantic overtures or sexual advances, infidelity, robbery, financial or property and other domestic disputes, etc.

Agents used

Any corrosive agent (mineral acids, organic acids and alkalis) and irritant plant juices, such as *Calotropis* may be used.

Target organ

Predominantly head and face. Other parts of the body may be involved.

Symptoms

Burns are deep and painless with blackening and charring of the affected areas. Ocular exposure often leads to blindness.

Complications

Blindness, scarring, disfiguration and deformities and infections.

Outcome

Serious physical as well as psychological trauma to the victim.

Cause of death

Death occurs from shock or toxemia in cases of extensive burns.

Treatment

- Ascertain the chemical involved. Remove the effected or contaminated clothing
- Irrigation (washing) of the affected parts and eyes copiously is the mainstay of treatment
- The affected areas are washed with plenty of water or sodium or potassium carbonate following which a thick paste of magnesium oxide or carbonate is applied
- Surgical reconstruction and repair may be required.

Note: Irrigation with water causes increased tissue penetration in carbolic acid exposure of skin, and hence, not recommended.

Preventive measures

- Restricted sale of acids. Over the counter sale of acids is discouraged
- Stricter penal provisions [in Indian Law, 326 A and 326 B are recently inserted to Section 326 Indian Penal Code (IPC) to deal with such cases stringently].

Medicolegal significance

- *Assault:* Preplanned and premeditated attempt to harm
- *Accidental spillage* is to be differentiated from intentional throwing of corrosive substances
- Blindness, and permanent disfiguration of the head or face, etc. amounts to *grievous hurt (Section 320 of Indian Penal Code)*
- *Section 326 of Indian Penal Code:* Corrosives are included as dangerous weapon or means in Section 326 of IPC (*For the purpose of Section 326 A and B IPC acid includes, any substance which has acidic or corrosive character or burning nature, capable of causing bodily injury leading to scars or disfigurement or temporary or permanent disability*).

Discuss carbolic acid poisoning in detail? Write a note on phenol marasmus, carboluria and ochronosis?

Carbolic acid poisoning is referred as *carbolism* and is characterized by strong *phenolic odor* in breath.

Carbolic acid (phenol) is rapidly absorbed on inhalation, ingestion and through skin and mucus membranes. Phenol is highly corrosive in nature and produces both local and systemic effects.

Clinical manifestations of acute poisoning

Local effects

- *Skin exposure:* Burning pain, numbness, blanching, severe burns and white opaque eschar formation. *Burns are painless.* Temporary or permanent blindness if eyes are involved
- *Ingestion:* Burning pain, irritation and inflammation of GI tract. Tongue is white and swollen
- *Inhalation:* Laryngeal and pulmonary irritation and edema.

Systemic effects

- *Central nervous system:* Central nervous system (CNS) depression, convulsions, coma, hypothermia, difficulty in breathing
- *Cardiovascular:* Features of shock
- *Renal:* Urine is scanty and dark (*carboluria*). Hematuria, albuminuria, oliguria or anuria may occur.

Chronic poisoning: It is associated with liver, kidney and ocular damage. Skin changes and oropharyngeal sores have been observed. Scanty or dark urine is a characteristic observation.

Signs and symptoms of carbolic acid poisoning can be summarized and remembered as (**mnemonic: *CARBOL***)*:*

- **C**orrosive effects, **C**arboluria, **C**onvulsions, **C**oma, **C**onstricted pupils, **C**yanosis
- **A**limentary tract: Gastrointestinal inflammation, pain in the throat and abdomen, nausea, vomiting, diarrhea, blood in vomitus and stools
- **R**enal insufficiency: Scanty dark green urine, decreased urine output
- **B**urns in the skin and oral cavity; **B**reath "phenolic"
- **O**ral ulcers, **O**chronosis, **O**cular involvement, characteristic **O**dor
- **L**ow BP, **L**ow urinary output.

Phenol marasmus (carbol marasmus)

Phenol marasmus refers to a disorder resulting from chronic inhalation of phenol that is characterized by anorexia, weight loss, weakness, headache, vertigo, muscle aches, dark urine and hyperpigmentation of the skin and sclera. Phenol marasmus was frequently reported as an occupational hazard among healthcare workers in the 19th century.

Carboluria

In carbolic acid poisoning; the urine turns dark or green on exposure to air commonly referred to as "carboluria". This greenish discoloration is attributed to the oxidation of the phenolic metabolites (*hydroquinone and pyrocatechol*) excreted in urine.

Ochronosis (carbolochronosis)

Ochronosis is characterized by hyperpigmentation in the cornea and various cartilages as a result of *chronic* exposure to phenols (hydroquinone). Hydroquinone gets deposited in the matrix of cartilage imparting a bluish gray appearance to the tissues.

Fatal dose

1–2 grams.

Fatal period

3–4 hours.

Treatment

- ABCD (maintain **a**irway, **b**reathing, **c**irculation, **d**econtamination) and symptomatic treatment
- Gastric lavage can be carried out without any risk of perforation as the gastric mucosa is leathery and thick in phenol poisoning.

Cause of death

- Central nervous system depression, toxic kidney damage.

Dermal exposure is shown to be fatal owing to its rapid absorption and systemic effects.

Postmortem appearances

- Corrosion of the skin; *leathery white and ash-gray* in appearance
- Tongue is usually white and swollen
- White necrotic lesions in the oropharynx and the GI tract (GIT)
- Phenolic odor from the mouth and in gastric contents
- The stomach mucosal folds appear grayish, thickened and leathery
- Pulmonary congestion and edema. Hemorrhagic nephritis is seen.

Medicolegal significance

Accidental exposure (including dermal contact) and suicidal ingestion of phenol is reported for its easy availability and its presence in the household as antiseptic and disinfectant. Its use in homicides is rare owing to its peculiar phenolic odor.

Write a short note on oxalic acid poisoning?

Oxalic acid (acid of sugar)

Oxalic acid is used as a beach, stain and ink remover.

Poisoning with oxalic acid produces both local and systemic effects.

- *Local effects* of oxalic acid poisoning are similar but milder to those seen in phenol poisoning.
- *Systemic effects* include hypocalcemia and renal damage that occur due to the affinity of oxalic acid to calcium ions in blood.

Clinical manifestations

Abdominal pain, vomiting (vomitus contains altered blood and mucus and has a *coffee ground* appearance), diarrhea, dilated pupils, features of tetany or hypocalcemia (muscle weakness, spasm and cramps), metabolic acidosis, oxaluria, oliguria or anuria (Flowchart 2).

Flowchart 2: Clinical manifestations of oxalic acid (OA) poisoning

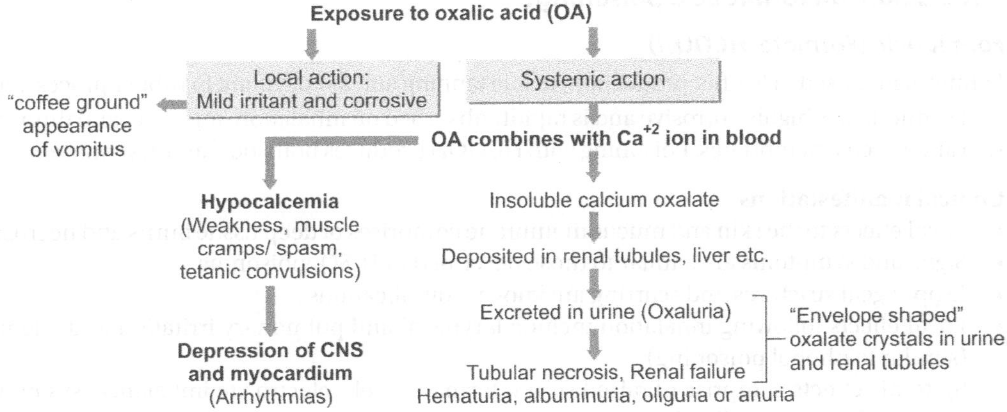

Abbreviation: CNS, central nervous system

Oxaluria

Oxaluria refers to excretion of ovoid or long needle shaped (picket fenced) monohydrate and envelope shaped or octahedral dihydrate calcium oxalate crystals in urine.

Fatal dose

15–30 grams.

Fatal period

1–2 hours.

Treatment

- Stomach wash with calcium lactate or gluconate, and symptomatic treatment
- Antidote in oxalic acid poisoning is calcium gluconate (slow IV administration of 10 mL of 10% calcium gluconate)
- Hemodialysis is recommended for management of acute renal failure.

Cause of death

Central nervous system depression, arrhythmias, toxic kidney damage or acute renal failure.

Postmortem appearances

- Congestion and corrosion of GI tract
- Scrapings from the mucosa may show the presence of calcium oxalate crystals
- Renal tubules are filled with oxalate crystals
- Organs are congested.

Note: Ingestion of ethylene glycol (an antifreeze agent) is the most commonly reported cause of OA poisoning. Ethylene glycol is metabolized to OA that is responsible for the toxic effects (For details, see Chapter no. 11 on Inebriants).

Oxalic acid is a constituent of few plants; its poisoning is reported following consumption of star fruit.

Write a note on formic acid poisoning?

Formic acid (Formate, HCOOH)

Formic acid is used in leather production, textile tanning and as coagulant in rubber processing.

Formic acid is highly corrosive and is rapidly absorbed on inhalation, ingestion and through skin and mucus membranes. Poisoning with HCOOH produces both local and systemic effects.

Clinical manifestations

- Local effects to the skin and mucus membrane comprises of deep tissue burns and necrosis
- Signs and symptoms are similar to those described in H_2SO_4 poisoning
- Esophageal strictures and scarring are known complications
- Local effects following inhalation include laryngeal and pulmonary irritation and edema (similar to phenol poisoning)
- Systemic effects comprise of raised serum formate levels, electrolyte imbalance, systemic acidosis, CNS and cardiac depression, intravascular, hemolysis, hematuria, and renal failure.

Treatment

- Decontamination. IV bicarbonates administered for correction of acidosis
- Folate therapy (for increased metabolism of HCOOH and its breakdown into nontoxic substances)
- Dialysis may be necessary in cases of severe toxicity.

Cause of death

Central nervous system depression, arrhythmias, toxic kidney damage or acute renal failure.

Postmortem appearances

Similar to those described in other corrosive acid poisonings.

Medicolegal significance

Mostly suicidal. Suicidal ingestion of formic acid is commonly reported from the state of Kerala (India) owing to its easy availability to individuals engaged in rubber plantation and production.

Note: Formate is a toxic metabolite formed in methanol poisoning that is responsible for its ocular toxicity.

Irritants: Nonmetallic Irritant Poisons (Phosphorus)

CHAPTER 6

Write a note on the properties of elemental phosphorus. Describe the clinical manifestations of acute phosphorus intoxication and its management. Mention the characteristic autopsy finding in fatal phosphorus poisoning and its medicolegal significance.

Two forms (allotropes) of phosphorus are white or yellow phosphorus and red phosphorus.

The characteristic features of the two varieties of phosphorus are listed in Table 1.

Table 1: Characteristic features of the two varieties of phosphorus

	White or yellow phosphorus (toxic)	*Red phosphorus (nontoxic)*
Uses	Insecticides (e.g. organophosphates) Rodenticides (e.g. zinc phosphide) Pesticides (e.g. aluminum phosphide) Firecrackers, gunpowder, explosives	Sides of the match box
Color	White or yellow	Red-brown
Odor and taste	*Garlicky*	Odorless and tasteless
Luminous	Yes, *glows in the dark*	No
Fuming	Yes, emits fumes on exposure to air	No
Inflammable	Yes, so preserved under water	No
Toxicity	Highly toxic	None

Note: Garlic odor is reported in phosphorus, organophosphates, thallium and arsenic poisoning. (**Mnemonic:** ***Garlicky odor POTA***)

Acute phosphorus (yellow) poisoning

Yellow phosphorus produces deleterious effects by its local as well as systemic action.

Mechanism of action

It is a protoplasmic poison that interferes with cellular oxidation.

Clinical manifestations of acute phosphorus intoxication

Clinical manifestations of acute phosphorus intoxication are described in three stages as illustrated in Table 2.

Table 2: Clinical manifestations of acute phosphorus intoxication

First stage	*Second stage*	*Third stage*
Stage of local toxicity *(0–3 days)*	*Symptom-free stage* *(next 2–3 days)*	*Stage of systemic toxicity* *Stage of recurrence after 2nd stage*
• *Ingestion:* Irritation of the GI tract, burning pain in throat and abdomen, nausea, vomiting and diarrhea • *Garlicky odor* in breath, vomitus and excreta • *Luminescent and smoking vomitus and diarrhea* is characteristic (***smoky or smoking stool syndrome***)	Stage of apparent recovery	• Nausea, vomiting, diarrhea, hematemesis and weakness • Hemorrhages in the skin, mucous membrane and viscera
		• *Hepatotoxicity:* Enlarged tender liver, jaundice, liver failure
		• *Renal toxicity:* Hematuria, oliguria, albuminuria and renal failure
• *Dermal contact:* Causes deep burns		• *Central nervous system:* Convulsions, delirium, coma

Abbreviation: GI, gastrointestinal

Fatal dose

60–120 mg.

Fatal period

2–8 days.

Treatment

- ABCD (maintain **a**irway, **b**reathing, **c**irculation, **d**econtamination) and symptomatic treatment
- Gastric lavage using potassium permanganate (1:5000 solution) as it oxidizes phosphorus to harmless phosphates. Gastric lavage is continued till garlicky odor disappears
- *Copper sulfate is a useful antidote* in phosphorus poisoning; it precipitates phosphorus into harmless copper phosphide. Its dose, however, needs to be monitored to prevent copper toxicity
- Activated charcoal can be used for adsorption of the poison
- No demulcents (oils and fats), as these dissolve phosphorus and increase its absorption
- Vitamin K therapy and blood transfusion to treat hypoprothrombinemia
- Peritoneal or hemodialysis in cases of acute renal failure.

Cause of death

- Shock and cardiovascular collapse in fulminant poisoning
- Central nervous system (CNS) depression, kidney or liver failure in acute intoxication.

Postmortem appearances

- 2nd to 3rd degree burns in cases of dermal contact
- Signs of jaundice (yellowish sclera and body tissues)
- Garlicky odor of stomach and bowel contents
- Luminous material in stomach and bowel
- Gastrointestinal (GI) tract is inflamed and congested with patchy corrosion and necrosis of gastric mucosa

- Hemorrhagic spots on the skin, mucous membrane and viscera (liver, lungs, kidney, heart, etc.)
- Yellow soft, enlarged, fatty and friable liver (*to be differentiated from acute yellow atrophy*)
- Respiratory tract inflammation and pulmonary edema.
- Other organs are congested.

Mnemonic: P4 (Phosphorus)
- **P**rotoplasmic poison
- **P**hotoluminescence
- **P**hossy jaw
- **P**urpuric spots

Medicolegal significance or circumstances of poisoning

- *Accidental poisoning:* Predominantly reported in children
- *Homicidal poisoning:* Delay in appearance of symptoms that are similar to acute liver diseases (*acute yellow atrophy of liver*) and its rapid oxidation favors the use of phosphorus containing compounds in homicides. The compound, however, needs to be mixed with alcohol or coffee to mask its typical odor and taste.
- *Arson:* White phosphorus in wet cloth cover is thrown on huts. As the cover dries, phosphorus being highly inflammable on exposure to air ignites, putting the hut on fire.

Write a note on "phossy jaw".

Phossy jaw (glass jaw)

Phossy jaw is the necrosis of the lower jaw in the region of decayed tooth due to inhalation of phosphorus fumes, hence, also referred as "phosphorus necrosis of the jaw".

It is an occupational hazard among workers in the match industry due to the chronic or long-term inhalation of the fumes of white or yellow phosphorus (Flowchart 1).

Flowchart 1: Phossy jaw in chronic phosphorus poisoning

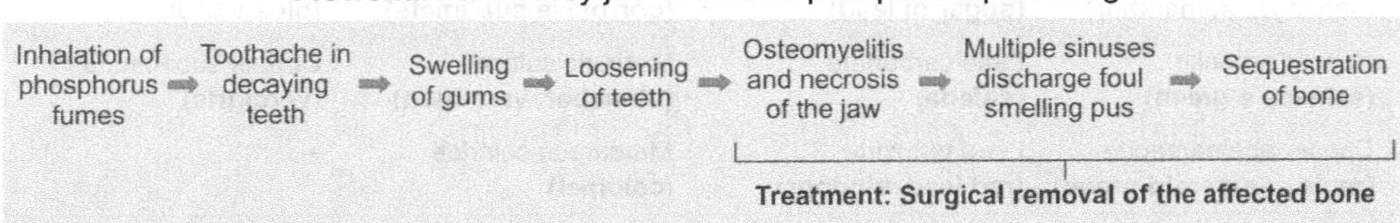

CHAPTER 7

Irritants: Metallic Poisons

List a few poisonous compounds of arsenic, lead, mercury and copper with their common names?

Metallic arsenic, mercury and copper are not absorbed from gastrointestinal (GI) tract and hence, nonpoisonous, while their salts are poisonous. On the other hand, metallic lead and its salts are poisonous. Toxic compounds of arsenic, lead, mercury and copper are listed in Table 1.

Heavy metals (elemental) per se have no/low toxicity; it is the metallic salts that are responsible for the toxic effects.

Table 1: Few poisonous compounds of arsenic, lead, mercury and copper with their common names

Arsenic (As)	*Lead (Pb)*	*Mercury (Hg)*	*Copper (Cu)*
Arsenic oxide or trioxide **(sankhya, somalkhar)**	Lead acetate **(sugar of lead)**	Mercuric chloride **(corrosive sublimate)**	Copper sulfate **(blue vitriol)**
Copper arsenite **(scheele's green)**	Lead carbonate **(safeda)**	Mercuric sulfide **(cinnabar, vermilion)**	Copper subacetate **(verdigris)**
Copper acetoarsenite **(paris or emerald green)**	Lead tetroxide **(red lead, sindoor)**	Mercurous chloride **(calomel)**	–
Arsenic acid, arsine gas	Lead chromate	Methyl mercury (organic)	–

Write a note on acute arsenic poisoning? Mention the differences between features of acute arsenic intoxication and cholera?

Acute arsenic poisoning

Mechanism of action

Arsenic combines with sulfhydryl (–SH) groups of mitochondrial enzymes and interferes with cellular oxidation by uncoupling of oxidative phosphorylation.

Clinical manifestations

Vary according to the type of poisoning:

- *Fulminant type:* Due to large doses. Death is rapid and due to shock. No GI symptoms.
- *Narcotic type:* Giddiness, formication, delirium, coma and death. Minimal GI symptoms.
- *Gastroenteric type:* Is the most common variant and resembles bacterial food poisoning.
  - *Gastrointestinal:* Symptoms are summarized in the Table 2.
  - *Liver:* Fatty infiltration

Table 2: Differences between acute arsenic intoxication and cholera

	Acute arsenic intoxication	Cholera
Temperature	Hyperthermia	Fever is rare
Taste	Metallic taste	None
Throat pain	Before vomiting	After vomiting
Vomitus	Contains mucus, bile and blood	Watery; no mucus, bile or blood
Diarrhea	After episodes of vomiting	Before vomiting
Stools	Rice watery and later bloody	Rice watery
Colic	Present	Absent
Tenesmus	Present	Absent
Conjunctiva	Inflamed	Not inflamed
Investigations	Electrocardiogram (ECG) changes Raised serum arsenic	Stool culture for *Vibrio cholerae*
Manner	Usually suicidal or accidental	Mostly accidental

- *Kidneys:* Oliguria, uremia, painful micturition
- *Cardiovascular:* Acute circulatory collapse, ventricular tachycardia and fibrillation
- *Central nervous system:* Hyperthermia, headache, vertigo, tremors, convulsions, coma
- *Skin:* Skin eruptions and delayed hair loss.

Fatal dose

0.1–0.2 grams of arsenic trioxide.

Fatal period

1–2 days.

Investigations

Blood and urine analysis, abdominal X-rays, electrocardiogram (ECG), complete blood count (CBC), liver function test (LFT) and renal function test (RFT).

Treatment

- Decontamination (gastric lavage and demulcents) and symptomatic treatment
- Chelation therapy with *British anti-lewisite* (BAL) or ethylenediaminetetraacetic acid (EDTA). Chelation is ineffective in arsine (gas) poisoning
- *Dimercaptosuccinic acid (*DMSA) (succimer) and penicillamine may be used alternatively.

Cause of death

- Shock and cardiovascular collapse in fulminant poisoning
- Dehydration, central nervous system (CNS) depression, kidney or liver failure in acute intoxication.

Postmortem appearances

- Features of dehydration such as cyanosis and sunken eyeballs, etc.
- Gastric mucosa is swollen and red (patchy or whole) especially in the pyloric region with lines of redness or submucus hemorrhages ***(red velvety appearance** or **velvety red congestion)***. ***Flea bitten appearance*** of the GI mucosa is said to be characteristic of arsenic poisoning.

- Brain is edematous and organs such as lung, liver, spleen and kidney are congested.
- ***Subendocardial petechial hemorrhages of the ventricles*** are characteristic autopsy observation in arsenic poisoning.

Write a note on acute lead and acute mercury poisoning?

Characteristic features of acute lead and acute mercury poisoning are shown in Table 3.

Table 3: Characteristic features of acute lead and acute mercury poisoning

	Acute lead (Pb) poisoning	*Acute mercury (Hg) poisoning*
Taste	Metallic taste	Metallic taste
Symptoms	Throat and abdominal pain, nausea, vomiting, diarrhea, oliguria/hematuria/albuminuria, fatigue, headache, convulsions and encephalopathy	• *Inhalation (Hg vapors):* ***Metal fume fever***, conjunctivitis, chest pain, dyspnea, pneumonitis, bronchiolitis, gingivitis, stomatitis, ***strawberry tongue***, loose teeth • *Ingestion (mercury salts):* Corrosion and gray-white coating of oral structures, throat irritation, hoarseness, breathing difficulty, GI distress, N+V+D (blood stained) with tenesmus. excessive salivation, glossitis, ulcerative gingivitis, loosening of teeth, AKI (proximal renal tubules necrosis)
Specific feature	*Black stools (lead sulfide)*	*Corrosive properties*
Death	Circulatory collapse	Circulatory collapse
Fatal dose	20–40 grams	1–4 grams
Fatal period	1–2 days	3–5 days
Treatment (GL, chelation and symptomatic including hemodialysis)	• GL (magnesium sulfate) • EDTA and BAL • Penicillamine • Hemodialysis • Symptomatic treatment	• GL (sodium bicarbonate) • BAL or EDTA, penicillamine • *BAL analogs:* DMSA (succimer), DMPS • Hemodialysis • Symptomatic treatment
Postmortem appearance	Patchy erosions of gastric mucosa, congested organs	Corroded and congested gastric mucosa. Congested organs, fatty liver
Associated syndrome	Fanconi's syndrome (affecting proximal renal tubules)	–

Abbreviations: AKI, acute kidney injury; BAL, *British anti-lewisite*; DMPS, *dimercaptopropanesulfonic acid; DMSA, dimercaptosuccinic acid; EDTA,* ethylenediaminetetraacetic acid; GI, gastrointestinal; GL, gastric lavage; N+V+D, nausea, vomiting and diarrhea

- Features of mercury poisoning resembles diphtheric colitis involving the ascending and transverse colon.

Note: Metal fume fever, also known as brass chills and monday morning fever results from inhalation of metal oxide vapors or fumes. It is characterized by fever, chills, headache, abdominal cramps, dyspnea, etc. Zn, Cu, Hg, Pb, Sb, etc. are the commonly involved metals. The recovery is spontaneous when the patient is kept away from the exposure.

Write a note on copper (Cu) poisoning?

Characteristic features of acute copper poisoning are shown in Table 4.

Table 4: Characteristic features of acute copper poisoning

Taste	*Metallic taste*
Symptoms	• Pain abdomen, nausea, vomiting, and diarrhea. Salivation, thirst, oliguria/hematuria/albuminuria, blue green secretions • *Severe cases:* Hemolysis, hemoglobinuria, jaundice, hypotension, convulsions, headache, difficulty in breathing • *Inhalation:* Sore throat and irritation • *Dermal exposure:* Contact dermatitis, green-blue skin
Specific symptoms	Increased salivation (***ptyalism***), blue or green vomitus
Death	Circulatory collapse, hepatic and/or renal failure
Fatal dose	15–30 grams
Fatal period	1–3 days
Treatment	• GL with 1% potassium ferrocyanide (antidote) • *Chelation therapy:* N-penicillamine, EDTA and BAL • Hemodialysis and symptomatic treatment
Postmortem appearance	Green-blue stomach contents, features of jaundice, congested gastric mucosa and organs
Associated conditions or syndromes	• Indian childhood cirrhosis (ICC) and Wilson's disease • Kayser-Fleischer ring is formed due to copper deposition in the cornea

Abbreviations: BAL, *British anti-lewisite; EDTA*, ethylenediaminetetraacetic acid; GL, gastric lavage;
Note: Chronic copper poisoning or copperiedus is characterized by blue or green line on gums, anemia, liver and kidney failure.

Write a note on chronic arsenic (As) poisoning?

Chronic arsenic poisoning

Chronic arsenic poisoning results from ingestion of its small doses over a period of time as an occupational hazard, taking contaminated food or water or due to its administration with homicidal intent.

Arsenic is a *cumulative poison* and is retained in bones, hair, nails and skin for years.

Manifestations of chronic poisoning appear in 2–8 weeks following ingestion.

Features of chronic arsenic poisoning can be remembered by the **mnemonic:** ***ARSENIC*** (features of acute poisoning are also listed in parentheses for easy remembrance)

- **A**ldrich-Mees' lines on nails (irregular thickening and bands of opacities), **A**nemia, **A**rsenophagist *(**A**cute renal failure in acute poisoning)*
- **R**ain drop pigmentation of skin (involving predominantly the flexures, face, neck, shoulders), **R**einsch's test *(**R**ice water stools and **R**habdomyolysis in acute poisoning)*
- **S**kin changes; Hyperpigmentation, hyperkeratosis of palms and soles *(**S**ubendocardial hemorrhages in acute poisoning)*
- **E**ncephalopathy
- **N**europathy (peripheral); sensory and motor involving all extremities, **N**ail changes: Aldrich-Mees' lines. **N**eutron activation analysis (NAA) for detection of arsenic
- **I**mbibition postmortem (cautious interpretation in cases of exhumation)
- **C**irrhosis, **C**hronic nephritis, **C**ardiac failure, **C**helation with BAL, **C**umulative poison *(**C**holera-like symptoms in acute poisoning)*.

Note: Postmortem imbibition of arsenic refers to imbibition (absorption) of arsenic from surrounding earth to the body or imbibition of arsenic from stomach to neighboring viscera.

Diagnosis

- History of chronic arsenic exposure and presence of characteristic signs and symptoms
- Reinsch's test, Marsh's test, atomic absorption spectroscopy (AAS) and neutron activation analysis (NAA) are employed to detect arsenic in body tissues, skin, hair, nails and bones, etc.

Treatment

Remove the patient from source of exposure. Chelation therapy with BAL.

Mention the medicolegal significance of arsenic poisoning with a note on "arsenophagists"?

Medicolegal significance or circumstances of arsenic poisoning

- *Accidental:* Intake of contaminated water or food, and non-judicious use of medicinal preparations.
- *Homicidal:* Arsenic qualifies as an ideal homicidal poison as the symptoms can be mistaken for cholera. Possibility of its detection in skin appendages, nails, hair, bones, and ashes, etc. after years, however, is a major disadvantage for its misuse

  Note: Analysis of the hair of Napoleon Bonaparte revealed high levels of arsenic raising the suspicion of chronic arsenic poisoning.
- *Abortifacients:* Arsenic pastes are used directly or on abortion sticks for procuring abortion
- *Carcinogenicity:* Arsenic has carcinogenic and teratogenic potential
- *Black foot disease*, an endemic peripheral vascular disease is associated with intake of arsenic from the artesian wells in regions of Taiwan
- *Postmortem imbibition of arsenic:* Interpretation of arsenic levels becomes significant especially in cases of exhumation
- *Arsenophagists:* These are individuals who take arsenic regularly as a tonic or aphrodisiac and develop tolerance to it. Such individuals can tolerate very high doses (up to 0.3 grams) of arsenic.

Write in detail about chronic lead (Pb) poisoning/Plumbism/Saturnism? Mention in brief the hematological changes in chronic lead poisoning?

Chronic lead poisoning

Features of chronic lead poisoning can be remembered by the **Mnemonic *ABCDEF or PB-LEAD***

Signs and symptoms

- **A**nemia [due to increased red blood cell (RBC) fragility and interference with hemoglobin synthesis], **A**menorrhea, **A**bortion, **A**lopecia and **A**norexia
- **B**asophilic stippling or punctate basophilia (clumps of ribosomes appear as dark blue spots in cytoplasm of RBCs during blood smear examination due to toxic action of lead on porphyrin metabolism) (basophilic—stained with basic dye; stippling—dotted appearance), **B**urtonian or **B**lue line on gums (lead line) at the junction of carious teeth (due to reaction of lead and hydrogen sulfide released from decaying food in mouth to form lead sulfide)

  Note: Blue line on gums may also be seen in mercury, copper and bismuth poisoning.
- **C**olic during night, **C**onstipation, **C**ircum-oral pallor, **C**oproporphyrin levels in urine (CPU) raised

- **D**rop (wrist drop and foot drop due to lead palsy; more common in adults, and in males)
- **E**ncephalopathy (lead encephalopathy is more common in children and is usually irreversible)
- **F**acial pallor (Earliest observed in the circum-oral region and occurs due to vasospasm).

Alternate mnemonic: *PB-LEAD*

- **P**allor, **P**lumbism, **P**ain colicky at night and constipation, **P**unctate basophilia
- **B**asophilic stippling or punctate basophilia, **B**urtonian or **B**lue line on gums (lead line).
- **L**ead palsy, **L**ead line on gums
- **E**ncephalopathy
- **A**nemia, **A**menorrhea, **A**bortion, **A**lopecia and **A**norexia
- **D**rop (wrist drop and foot drop).

Diagnosis

History of chronic exposure and presence of characteristic signs and symptoms.

Laboratory investigations

- Blood lead concentration 0.1–0.6 mg per 100 mL
- Zinc protoporphyrin and free erythrocyte protoporphyrin (FEPP) levels more than 50 mg/100 mL
- *Lead in urine:* 0.25 mg of lead/liter of urine
- Increased levels of CPU and aminolevulinic acid in urine (ALAU)
- *Peripheral blood smear:* Basophilic stippling (>200 affected cells/mm^3)
- *X-ray:* Transverse radio-opaque bands (lead lines) at metaphysis of long bones in children.

Treatment

- Remove the patient from source of exposure. Chelation with EDTA and BAL
- Alternatively, DMSA (succimer), 2,3-*dimercapto-1-propanesulfonic acid* (DMPS) or penicillamine can be given
- Magnesium or sodium sulfate (unabsorbed lead salts form insoluble lead sulfate and are excreted).

The hematological effects in chronic lead poisoning are described in Flowchart 1.

Flowchart 1: Hematological effects in chronic lead poisoning

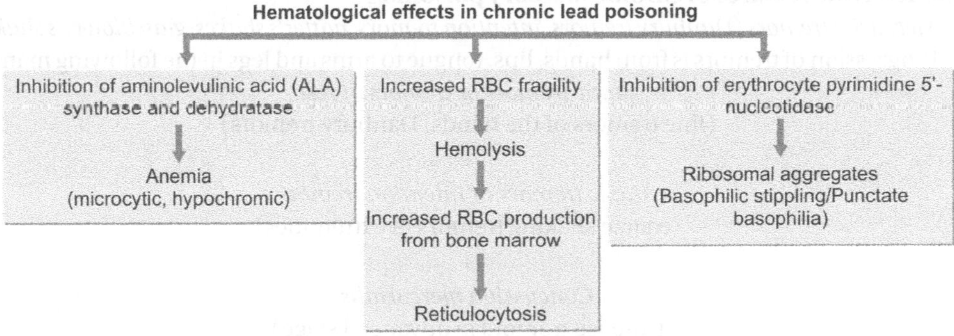

Abbreviation: RBC, red blood cell

Note: Lead inhibits enzymes aminolevulinic acid (ALA) dehydratase, coproporphyrinogen oxidase and ferrochelatase resulting in inhibition of heme synthesis

Mention the medicolegal significance of lead poisoning with a note on "lead ammunition and toxicity"?

Medicolegal significance or circumstances of lead poisoning

- *Accidental:* Poisoning due to intake of contaminated air/water/food
- *Pica:* Ingestion of paint fragments containing lead by children (the term "pica" in general refers to an appetite for nonfood substances, e.g. paper, hair, nail, lead containing paint fragments, etc.)
- Occupational exposure among painters is a cause of chronic lead toxicity.
- *Homicidal and suicidal:* Rare
- Abortifacient and cattle poison.

Lead ammunition and toxicity

- Retained lead bullets (*souvenir bullet*)/bullet fragments/pellets can cause lead toxicity over a period of time as lead gets slowly dissolved in body fluids
- Ingestion of lead bullets or meat (hunting) contaminated with lead fragments can cause toxicity
- Inhalation of lead dust in shooting ranges can result in increased lead levels and lead toxicity.

Write a note on chronic mercury (Hg) poisoning or hydrargyrism?

Chronic mercury poisoning

Features of chronic mercury poisoning by its various forms are summarized in Table 5.

Table 5: Features of chronic mercury poisoning

Mercury vapors	*Inorganic mercury compounds*	*Organic mercury compounds*
Triade of • ***Gingivostomatitis*** • ***Erethism*** • ***Tremors*** ***Mnemonic: GET***	Anorexia, weight loss, insomnia, tremors, *ptyalism* (hypersalivation), gingivitis, loosening of teeth, blue line in gums, impaired memory and intellect, renal damage, liver damage	Ataxia, tremors, sensory disturbances (hand and feet), constriction of visual fields, speech and auditory impairment, memory loss

Characteristic features of chronic mercury poisoning

- *Mercurial tremors (Danbury tremors, intention tremors, hatter's shakes, glassblower's shakes):* Progression of tremors is from hands, lips, tongue to arms and legs in the following manner:

Static tremors or tremors at rest
(fine tremors of the hands; Danbury tremors)
↓
Ataxic tremors or intention tremors
(coarse shaking tremors of extremities)
↓
Concussion mercurialis
(intense tremors in advanced stage)
Inability to perform routine tasks such as writing, walking, dressing, etc.

- *Mercurial erethism (erethism, neuropsychiatric manifestations, Mad Hatter):* Characterized by severe behavior and personality changes such as: emotional instability, timidity, shyness, irritability, excitability, anxiety, depression, insomnia, fatigue, social withdrawal, delusions, hallucinations, suicidal melancholia and manic depressive psychosis
- *Mercuria lentis (ocular changes in exposure to mercury vapors):* Brownish pigmentation (mercury deposition) on the anterior lens capsule, occurs bilaterally.
  - *Brown malt reflex* on slit lamp examination is characteristic
  - *Vision is not affected.*
- *Acrodynia (acro, extremity; dynia, pain):* Also known as pink disease, Feer disease, Swift's disease, erythroderma, etc.

  Acrodynia is an idiosyncratic hypersensitivity reaction in children that is characterized by:

  Painful, **p**ink, **p**uffy, **p**erspiring, **p**aresthetic, **p**eeling, **p**ruritic hands and feet, accompanied with **p**olyneuritis, **p**hotophobia, desquamating rashes, behavioral changes, insomnia, irritability, etc. The features of Pink disease can be remembered by the **mnemonic: 9Ps**

Features of chronic mercury poisoning are revised as **(mnemonic: *HG-MERCURI*):**

- **H**ydrargyrism, **H**atter's shakes
- **G**ingivostomatitis, **G**lassblower's shakes, **G**ums-blue lines
- **M**inamata disease, **M**ental deterioration, **M**ercuria lentis, **M**ercurial tremors
- **E**rethism, **E**ye changes (pigment deposition on anterior lens capsule)
- **R**enal changes (glomerular and tubular damage)
- **C**oncussion mercurialis, **C**erebral palsy in children
- **U**rticaria
- **R**ashes
- **I**diosyncratic hypersensitivity reaction (acrodynia), **I**ntention tremors.

Diagnosis
- History of chronic exposure and presence of characteristic signs and symptoms
- Raised mercury levels in blood and urine.

Treatment

Remove the patient from source of exposure. Chelation therapy with BAL and DMSA. Alternatively, D-penicillamine or DMPS can be given.

Mention the medicolegal significance of mercury poisoning with a note on "Minamata disease"?

Medicolegal significance or circumstances of mercury poisoning

- *Homicidal and Suicidal:* Rare
- *Accidental:*
  - Consumption of fishes containing organic mercury compounds like methyl mercury can result in poisoning (Minamata disease)
  - Mercury vapors from dental amalgam fillings especially during restorations or taking hot food can cause poisoning
- *Occupational exposure:* Mostly occurs due to inhalation of mercury vapors
  - *Dentists* are exposed to mercury vapors from dental amalgam

  - Mercury nitrate was used in *hat industries* and hatters (workers in hat industries) exposed to mercury fumes suffered from tremors (*hatter's shakes*) and neuropsychiatric symptoms (*mad as a hatter*)
  - Similarly, tremors observed in workers of *ornamental glass manufacturing units (Glassblower's shakes)*.

Note
- Dental amalgam is a mixture of silver, tin, copper and zinc set with mercury.
- Mercury ingested due to breaking of thermometer in mouth does not cause poisoning.
- Mercury thiocyanate was used in fireworks "Pharaoh's serpent" called Diwali snake in India.

Minamata disease (organic mercury poisoning)

Minamata disease (organic mercury poisoning) is described in Flowchart 2.

Flowchart 2: Organic mercury poisoning resulting in Minamata disease

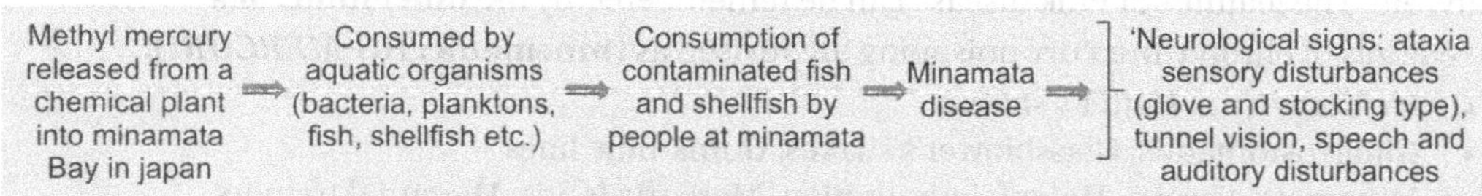

Write a note on thallium (Th) poisoning?

Characteristic thallium triad consists of the following manifestations **(mnemonic 3As)**
- **A**lopecia of sudden onset (loss of scalp hair, lateral part of eyebrows and eyelashes). Alopecia is the most *common* and presenting symptom in thallium poisoning
- **A**bdominal pain
- **A**scending peripheral neuropathy (*differential diagnosis: Guillain-Barré syndrome*). Other features include:
  - *Mees' line on nails* (similar to arsenic poisoning), dry scaly skin of palm and soles, and rashes
  - Behavior and personality changes, visual impairment, abnormal color vision, diplopia, and optic atrophy.
  - GI symptoms are minimal in chronic thallium poisoning.

Treatment

Gastric lavage with 1% potassium iodide. Prussian blue is the treatment of choice.

Medicolegal significance

Accidental, suicidal and homicidal poisonings are reported.

Note: Heavy metals (As, Pb, Hg, Th, etc.) get accumulated in skin, soft tissues, bones, hair, nails, etc. and can be detected even in the cremated remains or ashes.

CHAPTER 8

Irritants (Organic): Plant Poisons

Enumerate some plant irritants. Mention their common names, active principles, fatal dose and specific medicolegal significance?

Details of plant irritants are summarized in Table 1.

Table 1: Plant irritants, their common names, active principles, fatal dose and specific medicolegal significance

Plant	*Other names*	*Active principles*	*Fatal dose*	*Medicolegal issues*
Abrus precatorius	*Rati,* crab's eye, Indian liquorice, rosary pea, kunch, gunja, gunchi	Abrin, abrine, abraline, abric acid, abrussic acid	1–2 crushed seeds or 100–120 mg abrin	• *Suis/needles/ spikes* • Arrow poison • Cattle poison • Abortifacient • Conjunctivitis*
Ricinus communis	Arand, castor, mole bean	Ricin, Ricinine	8–10 crushed seeds or 6 mg ricin	• Abortifacient • Cattle poison • *Bioterrorism*
Croton tiglium	Jamalgota, Nepala	Crotin, crotonoside, crotonoleic acid	4–5 seeds or 2–5 mL oil	• Arrow poison • Abortifacient
Semecarpus anacardium	*Dhobi's nut, marking nut,* bhilawa	Bhilawanol, Semecarpol	6–8 seeds	• Vitriolage • Conjunctivitis* • Artificial bruise*
Calotropis gigantea	Akdo, madar, erukku	Calactin, calotoxin, calotropin, uscharin, *gigantin—most toxic*	–	• Abortifacient • Conjunctivitis* • Artificial bruise*
Calotropis procera	Sodom apple	Calactin, calotoxin, calotropin, uscharin	–	*Roots used as snake repellant*
Plumbago rosea	Lal chitra	Plumbagin	–	• Abortifacient • Artificial bruise*
Capsicum annuum	Chili, mirch	Capsaicin, capsicin	–	• *Hunan hand*** • *Hyderabadi goli#*

*Malingering: Fabricating symptoms for vested interests, e.g. Abrus seed dust or Semecarpus or Calotropis sap-induced conjunctivitis is produced intentionally to seek leave or application of irritant plant juices (Semecarpus, Plumbago, Calotropis) can produce lesions mimicking bruise referred to as artificial bruises in order to frame someone for causing injury.

**Hunan hand (Chilli burn): A painful contact dermatitis in those handling chili peppers with bare hands. It is an occupational hazard attributed to substance P released by capsaicin.

#Hyderabadi goli: A form of torture where police baton (lathi) smeared with chili powder is inserted in anus.

What is toxalbumin (Phytotoxins)? Name some toxalbumins.

Toxalbumins (tox refers to toxic and albumin refers to proteins) or phytotoxins (plant toxins).

- Toxalbumins are toxic proteins that inhibit protein synthesis by inactivating ribosomes and cause severe multiple organ system damage
- Toxalbumins cause hemagglutination and profound hemorrhage in severe cases
- These toxic properties resemble those of snake venom
- Abrin poisoning resembles viperine snake bite, while ricin is considered more poisonous than cobra venom
- There is no specific antidote for toxalbumin exposure. Gastric decontamination is beneficial
- Some of the toxalbumins are *abrin* (in *Abrus*), *ricin* (in *Ricinus*) and *crotin* (in *Croton*). These can be remembered by the **mnemonic:** ***ARC or CAR*** for **A**brin, **R**icin, and **C**rotin.

Describe the clinical manifestations of poisoning with plant irritants and its management?

- *Clinical manifestations* are the direct effects of irritation and vary as per the mode of entry
- *Local application (skin or mucosa):* Irritation, burning sensation, erythema, vesication
- *Ocular exposure (seed dust):* Reddening, lacrimation, conjunctivitis, temporary blindness.
- *Inhalation:* Sneezing, rhinorrhea, tightness of chest, bronchitis
- *Ingestion:* Throat irritation and pain, nausea, vomiting, diarrhea, pain abdomen, cramps
- *Injection (Abrin):* Oozing, inflammation, edema at the site of injection
- *Management:*
  - Treatment is symptomatic and supportive
  - Skin or eyes should be washed thoroughly with water
  - Gastric lavage in case of ingestion
  - Maintain fluid volume and electrolyte balance.

Note: Ingestion of intact seeds is harmless as they escape digestion due to the hard coat. Poisoning occurs when seeds are chewed or on ingestion of crushed seeds.

Write briefly on Ricinus communis poisoning?

The seeds of *Ricinus communis* contain a glycoprotein, ricin, which is regarded as the most potent phytotoxin. Ricin is released on chewing or crushing of seeds leading to poisoning.

Action

Ricin irreversibly inhibits protein synthesis through inhibition of ribonucleic acid (RNA) polymerase.

Clinical manifestations

- *Ingestion:* Digestive enzymes degrade ricin to a certain extent. Gastrointestinal symptoms (nausea, vomiting, diarrhea and abdominal cramps), dehydration and hypovolemic shock, hemolysis, hepatic and renal failure is observed
- *Inhalation:* It may be life-threatening. Respiratory irritation, cough, dyspnea, and rapid onset of flu-like symptoms including fever, weakness, nausea and myalgia are observed
- *Injection:* Pain and necrosis of the muscle at injection site
- *Dermal or ocular contact:* Allergic reactions are common. May cause conjunctivitis.

Treatment

Symptomatic and supportive.

Fatal dose

Ingestion of 8–10 crushed seeds.

Fatal period

Within 3–5 days.

Medicolegal significance

- *Accidental poisoning:* It occurs following consumption of castor seeds
- *Homicide:* A case is reported where a poisonous dart laced with ricin was fired from a concealed umbrella tip into the thigh of a Bulgarian national Georgi Markov in 1978 at a bus stop in London resulting in his death
- *Bioterrorism agent:* Ricin poses a potential threat as a weapon of mass destruction. A *ricin bomb* was developed by the British military during the Second World War.
- Castor oil is used as a lubricant and purgative. It contains ricinoleic acid, and is non-poisonous. *Castor oil* is extracted from castor bean on heating which inactivates ricin (heat labile). Ricin is present in the left over residues (press cake) during oil extraction process.

Note: Croton oil contains crotonoleic acid, and is poisonous, crotin is confined to press cake.

Write a short note on "Sui"?

Sui

Sui is also known as spikes or needles.

Suis are fine needles made of abrin which is used to kill cattle or for homicidal purposes.

Preparation of "Suis"

Abrus seeds are crushed into powder, and mixed with opium, onion and *Datura*. The mixture is made into a paste with spirit or water. Sharp, small needles (15 mm length and weighing nearly 100 mg) are then made from the paste and dried in the sun so that it becomes hard and ready to inject.

Principle

Abrin, a very potent toxalbumin is heat labile (destroyed on heating or boiling) and acid labile (inactivated by gastric juices). Its effects on ingestion are minimal but it is highly toxic when injected.

Method of injection

- A pair of suis is mounted on a wooden handle and shoved into the back of the cattle
- Sui may be held between fingers and the person is struck on the face, back or buttocks.

Clinical manifestations

(Resemble Viperine Snake Bite)

Localized pain, oozing of hemorrhagic fluid, inflammation, edema, ecchymosis, and necrosis at and around the site of injection. Drowsiness, vertigo, convulsions and death follows if untreated.

Management

- Needles (suis) and their fragments are dissected out, followed by symptomatic treatment.
- Injection antiabrin *(considered as specific treatment is no longer recommended).*

Fatal period

Death occurs in 3–5 days.

Medicolegal significance

Used as a weapon for killing humans and cattle. It is preferred as the puncture marks and symptoms resemble snake bite envenomation and the attacker may escape suspicion.

Differentiate between true and artificial bruise?

The major differences between true and artificial bruise is illustrated in Table 2.

Table 2: Differences between true and artificial bruise

No.	Feature	True bruise	Artificial bruise
1.	*Reason*	Trauma	Malingering
2.	*Causative action*	Blunt force or agent	Application of irritant juices
3.	*Site*	Anywhere on the body	Usually on the accessible areas
4.	*Shape*	Regular; corresponds to the inflicting weapon	Irregular
5.	*Margin*	Diffuse and irregular	Well-defined and regular
6.	*Erythema and inflammation*	At the site of trauma	In the surrounding areas
7.	*Itching*	Absent	Present
8.	*Vesication*	Absent	Present
9.	*Ulceration and sloughing*	Absent	Present
10.	*Color changes*	Color changes with healing	No color changes
11.	*Contents*	Extravasated blood	Acrid serum
12.	*Chemical tests*	Negative	Positive for toxic principles

Irritants (Organic): Animal Bites and Envenomation

CHAPTER 9

Comment briefly on the various venomous snakes and their families. Write a note on snake venom?

The various venomous snakes and their families are listed in Table 1.

Table 1: Common venomous snakes and their families

Family	*Elapidae*	*Viperidae*		*Colubridae*	*Hydrophidae*
Subfamily		*Viperinae*	*Crotalinae*		
Snakes	Cobra	Russell's viper	Pit vipers	Asian rat snake	Sea snakes
	Krait	Saw-scaled viper	Rattle snakes	Tree snake	

Note

- Viper bites are the most common venomous snake bites on humans globally.
- Colubridae is the largest snake family, mostly non-venomous and non-harmful to humans.

Snake venom

The venom is modified saliva, injected through grooved and hollow or canalized fangs. It is a mixture of many toxic proteins and enzymes such as neurotoxins, cardiotoxins, hemolysins, ophioxidases, cholinesterases, phosphatases, nucleotidases, hyaluronidase, etc.

Based on the nature of venom, snakes can be classified as shown in Table 2.

Table 2: Classification of snakes based on the nature of venom

Nature	*Neurotoxic*	*Vasculotoxic (hemotoxic)*	*Myotoxic*
Family	Elapidae	Viperidae	Hydrophidae
Snakes	Cobra, krait	Vipers	Sea snakes
Cause of death	Respiratory paralysis	*Disseminated intravascular coagulation* (DIC), renal failure	Renal or hepatic failure

Note

- Venoms do not cause toxicity if ingested as these are not absorbed through intact gastrointestinal (GI) mucosa.

List some of the venomous snakes commonly found in India. Mention the differences between venomous and nonvenomous snakes, and mention some distinct identification features of venomous snakes found in India?

Common venomous snakes found in India are described in Table 3.

Table 3: Common venomous snakes found in India (See chapter 26 for pictures of snakes)

Cobra	*Krait*	*Viper*
Common cobra (nag, spectacled cobra) *Naja naja*	Common krait *Bungarus caeruleus*	Russell's viper *Daboia or Vipera russelii*
King cobra (rajnag or nagraj) *Ophiophagus hannah*	Banded krait *Bungarus fasciatus*	Saw-scaled viper *Echis carinatus*

Note

- "The big four" important snake species in India are common cobra (N. naja), common krait (B. caeruleus), Russell's viper (D. russelii) and saw-scaled viper (E. carinatus).

At times killed or live snakes are brought to the emergency room along with the victim of snake bite to find if the snake was venomous or not, and to specifically identify the snake species, if possible.

Venomous and nonvenomous snakes can be differentiated based on the features that are illustrated in Fig. 1 and described in Table 4.

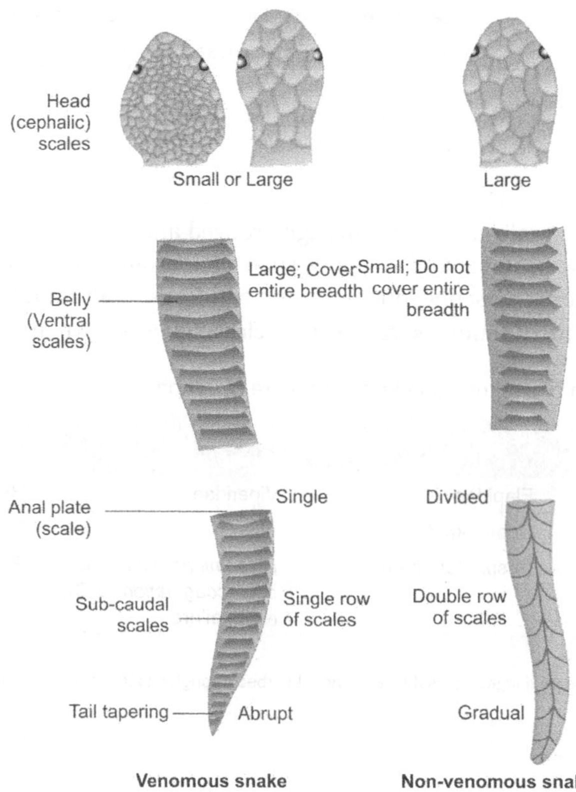

Fig. 1: Identifying features; venomous versus non-venomous snakes

Table 4: Differences between venomous and nonvenomous snakes

Venomous snakes	Identifying features	Nonvenomous snakes
Large (cobra, krait), small (viper)	**Head scales**	Large
Large (covers the entire breadth)	**Belly scales (ventral)**	Small (do not cover the entire breadth)
Divided	**Caudal scales**	Not divided
Rounded (flat in sea snakes)	**Tail**	Rounded
Short (cobra, krait), long (viper)	**Fangs (hollow)**	None
Usually in a single row	**Teeth (short and solid)**	In multiple rows
Mostly nocturnal	**Habitat**	Diurnal or nocturnal

Identifying features of common venomous snakes is described in Flowchart 1 and shown in Fig. 2.

Flowchart 1: Identifying features of common venomous snakes

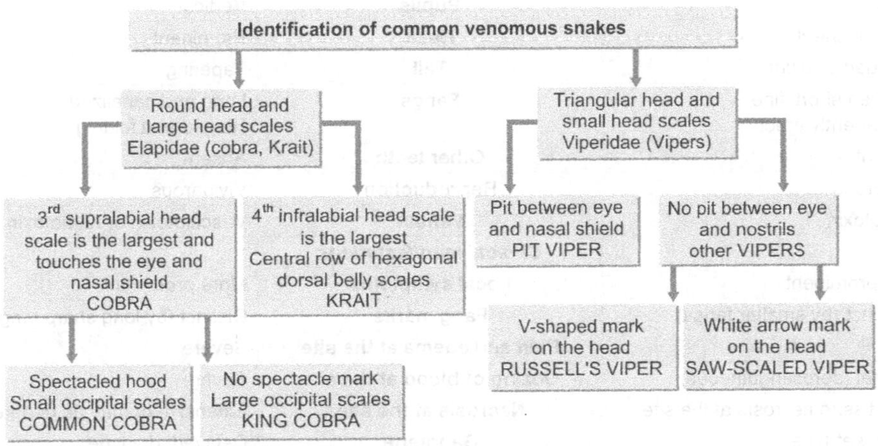

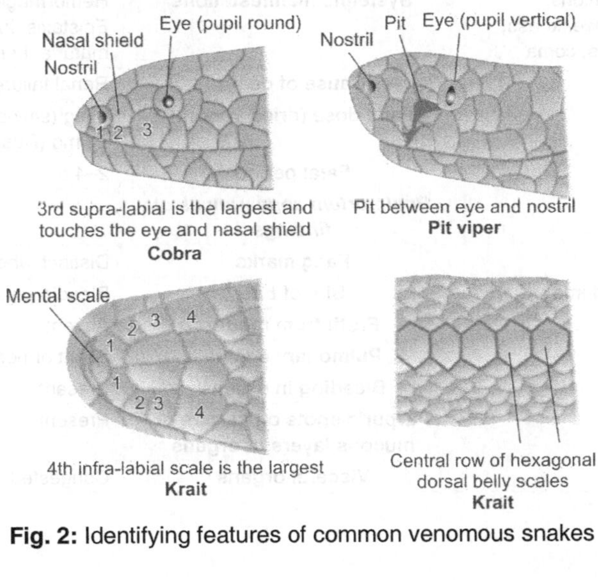

Fig. 2: Identifying features of common venomous snakes

Describe the morphology of Cobra and Viper, and the clinical manifestations and postmortem findings observed in cobra and viper envenomation?

Morphology of cobra and viper along with clinical manifestations and postmortem findings in cases of their envenomation are described in Table 5 in a easy to remember comparative format for the ease of readers.

Table 5: Morphology of snake, clinical manifestations and postmortem findings in cobra and viper envenomation

Cobra	*Differentiating features*	*Viper*
	Morphology	
Smaller, globular	**Head**	Larger, triangular
Spectacle mark in cobra	**Mark on the head**	V-shaped or white arrow mark
Large (3rd supralabial largest)	**Head scales**	Small (large with pit in pit viper)
Circular	**Pupils**	Vertical
Not prominent	**Neck**	Prominent
Rounded or blunt	**Tail**	Tapering
Grooved short, fine Permanently erect	**Fangs**	Long and canalized Hinged and folding
Present	**Other teeth**	Absent
Oviparous	**Reproduction**	Viviparous
Neurotoxin	**Venom**	Vasculotoxin or hemotoxin
	Clinical manifestations	
Less prominent	**Local symptoms**	More prominent
Indistinct (by smaller fangs)	**Fang marks**	Distinct (by long sharp fangs)
Mild	**Pain and edema at the site**	Severe
Minimal (serosanguineous)	**Oozing of blood at the site**	Severe
Early tissue necrosis at the site	**Necrosis at the site**	Extensive or may be gangrenous
Early, wet type	**Gangrene**	Delayed, dry type
Neurologic manifestations: Drowsiness, muscle weakness, paralysis, convulsions, coma	**Systemic manifestations**	Hemorrhagic manifestations: Epistaxis, bleeding of gums, hematuria, hematemesis, (DIC)
Respiratory failure	**Cause of death**	Renal failure or hemorrhage
12 mg (king cobra) 15 mg (cobra)	**Fatal dose (dried venom)**	8 mg (saw-scaled viper) 20 mg (Russell's viper)
30 minutes–1 day	**Fatal period**	2–4 days
	Postmortem appearances or findings	
About 1.25 cm deep	**Fang marks**	Distinct, about 2.5 cm deep
Slight oozing, mild edema	**Site of bite**	Bleeding, swelling and necrosis
Present	**Froth from mouth**	Absent
Prominent	**Pulmonary edema**	Slight or none
Absent	**Bleeding in organs**	Present
Absent	**Purpuric spots on serous or mucous layers of organs**	Present
Congested	**Visceral organs**	Congested

Describe the clinical manifestations and severity of snake bite envenomation. Write a note on management of snake bite envenomation?

Clinical manifestations

Clinical manifestations depend on the following factors:

- *Victim related:* Severe in children (*age*), malnourished (*nutritional status*) and in those with increased *sensitivity* to venom. *Physical activity* increases the rate of spread of venom and its severity.
- *Snake related:* Severity depends on the *snake species* and *amount of venom* injected.

Note: About 20% of the venomous snake bites are dry bites, i.e. no venom is injected in the bite.

- *Bite related:* Severity is more in bites on the head and face than on extremities (*location*), bites deep into the vessels (*depth*) and in cases of multiple bites (*number of bites*).

Clinical manifestations of cobra bite envenomation (Neurotoxic effects)

- *Local:* Fang marks, pain at bite site, mild edema, serosanguineous discharge or oozing of blood from the bite site, blistering and early tissue necrosis at the site, lymphangitis, and tender and enlarged regional lymph nodes
- *Systemic:* Nausea, vomiting, headache, vertigo, hypersalivation, drowsiness, muscle weakness and paralysis. Paralysis of the extremities which extends to the trunk and head resulting in drooping of head (*broken neck sign* due to the paralysis of the neck muscles), dysphagia, dysarthria, drooping of lower lip and frothing from mouth, *ptosis (one of the most common and early sign)* due to involvement of extraocular muscles, external ophthalmoplegia, etc. Respiration is shallow and labored due to respiratory or diaphragmatic muscle paralysis followed by convulsions, coma and death.

Clinical manifestations of krait bite envenomation (Neurotoxic effects)

- *Local:* Minimal (invisible fang marks, minimal or no pain and no edema at the site of bite)
- *Systemic:* Similar but milder than cobra. No nausea, frothing or convulsions are observed. Victim often complaints of abdominal cramps. Drowsiness is more marked.

The possibility of krait bite should be considered in sudden onset of neuroparalytic features in an otherwise healthy individual.

Clinical manifestations of viper bite envenomation (Vasculotoxic or hemotoxic effects)

- *Local:* Distinct fang marks, severe pain at bite site, gradually progressing edema, localized bleeding, ecchymosis, erythema, blistering with extensive tissue necrosis and gangrenous changes at times, lymphangitis, and tender and enlarged regional lymph nodes.
- *Systemic:* Bilateral parotid swelling *(viper head)*, subconjunctival hemorrhages, epistaxis, bleeding of gums, hemoptysis, hematemesis, rectal bleeding, hematuria and *disseminated intravascular coagulation* (DIC). DIC may cause hemoglobinuria and acute renal failure. Headache, dizziness and respiratory depression may occur. Intracranial (subarachnoid) and retroperitoneal or intraperitoneal hemorrhages, tachycardia, hypotension and death due to hemorrhagic shock.

Fatal dose

6 mg (*krait*), 12 mg (*king cobra*), 15 mg (*cobra*), 8 mg (*saw-scaled viper*), 20 mg (*Russell's viper*) of dried venom.

Fatal period

30 minutes to 1 day (cobra), 1–2 days (krait), 2–4 days (viper).

Snake venom ophthalmia/venom ophthalmia/cobra spit ophthalmia

Snake venom ophthalmia refers to ocular manifestations of "spat" venom (venom spat into the eyes) by the spitting elapids or other snakes. Local spread of venom may affect the 7th cranial nerve. Symptoms include severe burning pain, profuse lacrimation with whitish discharge, swollen eyelids, photophobia and temporary blindness. Corneal ulceration, corneal scarring and permanent blindness are also reported with some species. Prompt decontamination by washing the eyes with plenty of water and symptomatic treatment with topical antibiotics and antihistamines is useful.

Management of snake bite envenomation

The management of snake bite envenomation is detailed as follows:

- Snake bite is a medical emergency; the victim of snake bite hence, requires urgent attention
- Identification of the snake species causing the bite is significant in its management. The offending snake can be identified by examination of the snake and/or the clinical manifestations of envenomation
- The management varies based on the clinical manifestations following the snake bite and the severity of envenomation. Assessment of the severity is vital in management of snake bites as shown in Table 6.
- Neurotoxic venom is known to cause early death so prompt diagnosis based on history and neurological examination is of utmost importance
- In case of viper bite (hemotoxic venom) deranged coagulation profile has diagnostic importance.

Table 6: Assessment of the severity of envenomation

Clinical manifestations	*Mild envenomation*	*Moderate envenomation*	*Severe envenomation*
Local (edema, erythema or ecchymosis)	Confined to the site of bite (within 7.5 cm)	Beyond the site (involves major part of the limb)	Involves the entire part and beyond (>100 cm from the site)
Systemic signs and symptoms	None	Nonlife-threatening (nausea, vomiting, weakness, mild tachypnea, tachycardia or mild hypotension, etc.)	Life-threatening (altered sensorium, respiratory distress, marked tachycardia or hypotension)
Coagulation profile	Normal	Mild derangement No significant bleeding	Markedly abnormal with severe bleeding
Management	*No antivenom*	*Antivenom therapy*	*Antivenom therapy*

Note: Envenomation is generally ruled out in absence of fang marks, pain, oozing of blood and edema at the site of bite and if the victim does not complaint of drowsiness or weakness within 30 minutes to few hours of the bite.

Immediate care or first aid

- Reassurance to relieve fright and fear is important, or the victim may die of psychological or neurogenic shock

Note: 3/4th snake bites are by nonvenomous snakes and do not require any specific treatment.

- Immobilization of the patient especially the affected part (to minimize the spread of venom)
- Shift the victim to the hospital for specific treatment. Say ***NO*** to the following:
  - No incision and suction of wound (can result in secondary infection and necrosis)
  - No tourniquet (inappropriately applied or too tight tourniquet can lead to gangrene)
  - No cryotherapy (causes tissue ischemia and increased possibility of tissue necrosis).
  - No application of herbs, "snakestones", etc. on the site of bite.

Specific treatment in snake bite envenomation

Antivenom therapy is the *specific antidote or treatment of choice* for snake envenomation.

In cases of moderate or severe envenomation (*See* Table 6), antivenom therapy should be started promptly. The antivenom should be administered by *slow intravenous (IV) injection or infusion.*

Dose

Recommended average initial dose is 10–20 vials for common krait, 10–20 vials for common cobra, 10 vials for Russell's viper and 5 vials for saw-scaled viper.

Each vial of freeze-dried (lyophilized) antivenom is reconstituted, with sterile water (10 mL) for slow IV injection (not more than 2 mL per minute) or given as slow IV infusion of reconstituted 50–100 mL antivenom in 250–500 mL isotonic saline or 5% dextrose.

The dose of antivenom is similar in children and adults.

Each vial of antisnake venom (ASV) is capable of neutralizing 6 mg of cobra venom, 6 mg of Russell's viper venom and 4.5 mg each of saw-scaled viper and common krait venom.

(**Note:** Indiscriminate use of antivenom is strongly discouraged owing to the life-threatening immune reactions associated with antivenom therapy).

- Antivenom can be monovalent (neutralizes the venom of a particular snake species) or polyvalent (neutralizes the venom of a group of snake species)
- Whenever possible (based on the availability of antivenom and identification of offending snake), monovalent therapy is preferred over polyvalent therapy. Snake venom detection kit is often used to decide on the antivenom to be administered
- In India, monovalent antivenom are not available, and polyvalent antivenom (ASV) serum (derived from equine or horse) is administered in cases of snake bite envenomation. Polyvalent ASV is effective against the four common venomous snake species found in the region (cobra, krait, Russell's viper, saw-scaled viper) and hence, even in absence of positive identification of the snake, *ASV therapy is started in moderate or severe envenomation* (*See* Table 6)
- *Antivenom reactions:* Antisnake venom therapy (antivenom therapy) has associated risks of life-threatening immune reactions (antivenom reactions). Antivenom reactions can be *Type I hypersensitivity* (immediate hypersensitivity) reactions occurring within few hours of initiating the treatment or *Type III hypersensitivity* (delayed hypersensitivity or serum sickness) reactions that are dose related and are reported in 1–10 days' time. Medical practitioners thus, should be cautious while administering ASV therapy. In the event of immediate anaphylactic reactions, ASV therapy should be transiently discontinued and adrenalin should be given urgently. For treatment of delayed reactions, antihistamines and corticosteroids are given. Skin and conjunctival hypersensitivity testing is not recommended as these cannot predict the immune reactions to antivenom. Antivenom reactions cannot be prevented by any treatment.

Supportive or ancillary treatment

- Clear the airways and start artificial ventilation to treat respiratory failure especially in elapid bites
- Transfusion of clotting factors and platelets or fresh whole blood if these are unavailable to combat hemostatic derangements in viper bites
- Treat hypotension and shock with colloid or crystalloids and atropine
- Dialysis is done in cases of acute kidney injury (AKI) and acute renal failure (ARF)
- Anticholinesterase [e.g. neostigmine intramuscular (IM)] along with atropine is found to be useful in patients with neurotoxic symptoms (*Tensilon test*: IV atropine is followed with IM neostigmine to check for any improvement in neuromuscular transmission before using this treatment)
- Tetanus prophylaxis and broad spectrum antibiotics to combat infections
- Fasciotomy for intracompartmental syndrome when intracompartmental pressure is more than 40 mm Hg
- Heparin is ineffective and is *not* recommended as it may cause bleeding.

Ophitoxemia (toxicity following snake bite envenomation) and its management are summarized in Flowchart 2.

Flowchart 2: Ophitoxemia and its management

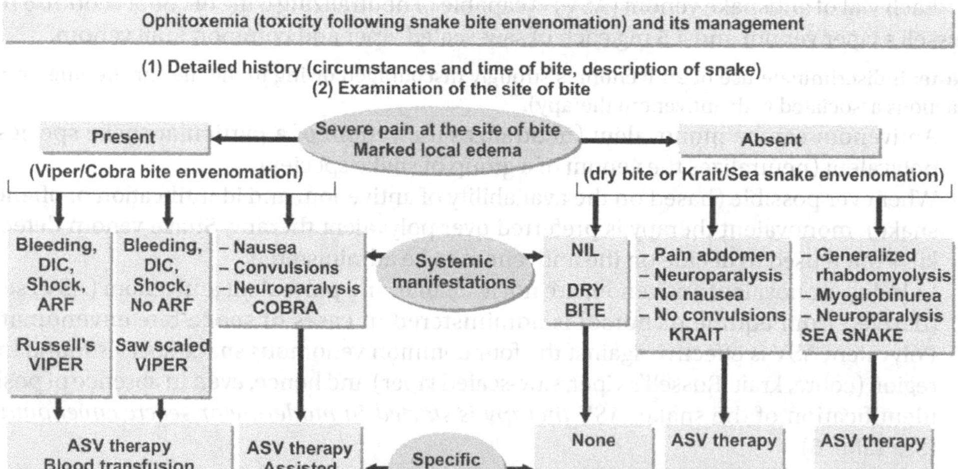

Abbreviations: ARF, acute renal failure; ASV, antisnake venom; DIC, disseminated intravascular coagulation

Note: Dry bite refers to snake bite where no venom is injected into the victim.

Mention the medicolegal implications of snake bite envenomation?

Medicolegal importance and circumstances of poisoning

- *Homicides:* These are rare. There are cases of snakes left on the sleeping unalarmed victims. Though a rare phenomenon, cases of injecting snake venom to cause death are also reported
- *Suicides:* These are very rarely reported in literature (It is reported that Queen Cleopatra committed suicide by snake bite)

- *Cattle poison:* Snakes or snake venom can be used as a cattle poison
- *Occupational hazard:* Most of the snake bite cases are accidental and reported in farming community, and in rural areas. Snake bite hence, is often considered as an occupational hazard
- *Financial compensation:* There are provisions for financial compensation to snake bite survivors for the injury caused, and to their kin in case of fatality. At times, false claims of snake bite are put by the victims or relatives for financial gains
- *Allegations of medical negligence* arise in deaths from antivenom immune reactions. Relatives often cite inappropriate therapy, lack of care or blood transfusion mismatch as the cause of death.
- *Autopsy:*
  - In case of death following snake bite, postmortem needs to be performed (Postmortem appearances are already described in Table 5). At autopsy, skin and underlying tissues around the alleged site of bite or fang marks and a control sample from another healthy site are dissected out, and preserved in saturated solution of common salt along with blood preserved in sodium fluoride solution and sent for analysis at the Regional Forensic Science Laboratory (RFSL).
  - Detection of snake specific antigens in the samples from the site of bite, serum, or urine by enzyme immunoassay or radioimmunoassay is confirmatory.

Write briefly on scorpion sting envenomation?

Scorpion (Mesobuthus tamulus) has a segmented tail with a venomous stinger at its end. Scorpion venom contains various toxins including neurotoxin (most potent), cardiotoxin, nephrotoxin, vasculotoxin histamine, serotonin, hyaluronidases, phosphodiesterases, etc.

The effects of venom are predominantly neurotoxic.

- *Action:* Predominantly on Na^+ channels causing prolonged neuronal activity (autonomic storm)
- *Clinical manifestations:* In humans vary with the scorpion species and age and nutritional status of the victim, etc. These may range from local skin reactions to life-threatening systemic effects
- *Local:* Pain, swelling and erythema
- *Systemic:* Paralysis, arrhythmias, respiratory depression, seizures, coma, etc.
- The characteristic features of scorpion sting envenomation can be remembered by the **mnemonic: *SCARPEAN***
  - **S**welling, **S**alivation, **S**wallowing difficulty, **S**eizures, **S**hock, **S**corpion antivenom (SAV) as treatment
  - **C**oagulopathy, **C**onvulsions, **C**oma, **C**erebral infarction and **C**erebral thrombosis
  - **A**llergy or anaphylaxis, **A**rrhythmias
  - **R**espiratory failure, **R**estlessness
  - **P**ain, ***P**riapism*, **P**ulmonary edema, **P**aralysis, **P**upils dilated, **P**ancreatitis, **P**razosin therapy
  - **E**ncephalopathy, **E**rythema
  - **A**utonomic storm, **A**ntivenom therapy
  - **N**eurotoxin, Na^+ channel mediated neuronal activity, **N**ystagmus

- *Treatment*
  - Immobilization of the limb and application of pressure bandage. Tetanus prophylaxis
  - Simultaneous administration of scorpion antivenom IV and prazosin orally is effective therapy
  - Symptomatic and supportive care (atropine, analgesics, antihistamines, barbiturates, etc.).
- *Cause of death:* Overall mortality is low. Death is due to respiratory or cardiovascular failure
- *Medicolegal significance:* Most of the cases are accidental, involving hands and feet.

Write a note on hymenoptera (bee and wasp) sting envenomation?

Bees and wasps are the winged insects of Hymenoptera group.

Stinger venom of these insects contains dopamine, histamine and neurotoxic enzymes, etc.

- *Clinical manifestations:* Depend on the number of stings and show individual variations. These range from local skin reactions to life-threatening anaphylaxis in sensitive individuals
- *Local:* Local skin reactions (pain, swelling and erythema)
- *Systemic:* Anaphylactic reactions (IgE-mediated) are usually associated with multiple stings. Nausea, vomiting, wheezing, hypotension, faintness, respiratory distress and unconsciousness may occur in cases of multiple stings
- *Treatment:* Wound care (removal of the stinger and cold compress), tetanus prophylaxis, adrenalin to combat anaphylaxis, and symptomatic and supportive treatment
- *Cause of death:* Airway obstruction or respiratory failure
- *Medicolegal significance:* Most of the cases are accidental.

Write a short note on Cantharides?

Cantharis vesicatoria/spanish fly/blister beetle

- *Active principle:* Cantharidin, which is highly irritant and readily absorbed through skin and mucosa. Cantharidin is present in the dried crushed insect (grayish powder with shiny green particles)
- *Action*
  - *Local:* Irritant
  - *Remote:* Nephrotoxic.
- *Clinical manifestations*
  - *Local:* Irritation, burning sensation, erythema, vesication or *blister formation* on the skin and involvement of oral mucosa, tongue, etc. when ingested
  - *Systemic:* Nausea, vomiting, burning sensation in the mouth and throat, dysphagia, dysarthria, pain abdomen, bloody diarrhea, renal toxicity (dysuria, oliguria, hematuria), *priapism in males and abortion in females*, convulsions, coma, death.
- *Management:* Treatment is symptomatic and supportive
- *Cause of death:* Renal failure
- *Postmortem appearances*
  - Presence of vesicles on skin and oral mucosa
  - Gastrointestinal mucosa is hemorrhagic with ulcerations and adherent shiny greenish particles of crushed fly
  - Organs are congested (pulmonary edema, renal hemorrhages).
- *Medicolegal significance or circumstances of poisoning*
  - Poisoning is often accidental owing to its use as a counter-irritant
  - Accidental poisoning occurs when used as an aphrodisiac or abortifacient (criminal abortion)
  - Rarely a cause of homicides and suicides.

CHAPTER 10

Neurotoxics: Somniferous Agents

Write a note on opium, its alkaloids, opiates and opioids. Describe the mechanism of toxicity, clinical manifestations and management of opium poisoning. Mention the postmortem findings and circumstances of opium poisoning.

Opium (Afim)

It is the dried latex obtained from the capsule of unripe opium poppy (*Papaver somniferum*). Incisions (lancing) are given on the unripe green capsule through which white latex oozes out. The latex is air-dried (dark brown) and scraped to obtain opium (crude opium).

Note: Ripe poppy capsule is dry and brown, and contains very small quantities of opium.

Around 25 different types of alkaloids are obtained from crude opium. These are grouped as:

Phenanthrene alkaloids/derivatives	*Benzylisoquinoline alkaloids/derivatives*
Morphine* (10%) Codeine (0.5%) and Thebaine (0.3%)	Papaverine (1%) Noscapine or Narcotine (6%)

*Principle alkaloid of opium is morphine.

Concentration of morphine in opium varies. It ranges between 9% and 14% in the Indian variety. Standardization of opium is done at the Government factory in Ghazipur such that the opium contains 10% morphine, and is referred as "standardized opium" or "*Ghazipur opium*".

Opiates

Derived from opium alkaloids, e.g. heroin (diacetylmorphine), apomorphine, etc.

Opioids

Opiate-like activity, but not derived from opium, e.g. pethidine, methadone, etc.

Note: *Poppy seeds* in the poppy capsule, known as *khas khas* or *posto* seeds are *nontoxic*, and often considered nutritious. These are commonly added to food items and especially used in bakeries.

Mechanism of action

Morphine has site specific depressant and stimulant action on the central nervous system (CNS). It acts on opioid receptors (μ, κ and λ) in the brain and has both depressant and stimulant effects (Table 1).

Table 1: Depressant and stimulant effects of morphine

Depressant effects	*Stimulant effects*
Analgesia, sedation and calming effects	*Chemoreceptor trigger zone (CTZ)*: Nausea and vomiting
Respiratory center: Decreased respiratory rate	*Oculomotor center*: Miosis (constricted pupils)
Cough center: Cough suppressant	*Vagal center*: Bradycardia
Temperature regulatory center: Hypothermia	*Certain cortical area and hippocampal cells*: Muscle rigidity and convulsions
Vasomotor center: Fall in blood pressure (BP)	

Other effects

Vasodilatation, bronchoconstriction, constipation, difficulty in micturition.

Clinical manifestations of acute poisoning

Clinical manifestations of acute poisoning are described in three stages (Table 2).

Table 2: The three stages of clinical manifestations of acute morphine poisoning

I: Excitement or euphoria	*II: Stupor or depression*	*III: Narcosis or coma*
Sense of well-being, talkativeness, flushing	Headache, nausea, vomiting, drowsiness	Muscles are relaxed, reflexes are absent. Secretions are diminished
Hallucinations	Constricted pupils	Subnormal temperature, low BP
Tachycardia, palpitations	Bradycardia, slow respiration	Respiratory depression

Fatal dose

Opium: 2 grams, morphine: 0.2 grams (oral) or 0.1 grams (parenteral).

Fatal period

6–12 hours.

Management

- Secure airways and assisted respiration. Oxygen therapy and suction of airways to clear the froth
- Gastric lavage with 1:5000 potassium permanganate ($KMnO_4$) solution as it oxidizes opiates.

  Note: Gastric lavage is useful even in delayed cases or when morphine was taken parenterally for the following reasons:
  - Resecretion of morphine can occur in stomach after absorption or in parenteral administration
  - Constipation and sphincter constriction may cause delayed gastric emptying.
- *Specific antidote:* Intravenous (IV) *naloxone*. Alternatively, IV *nalorphine* may be administered
- Supportive and symptomatic treatment for convulsions (diazepam), hypotension (vasopressors), pulmonary edema (diuretics), fluid and electrolyte imbalance, etc.

Cause of death

Respiratory failure.

Postmortem appearances

The major postmortem appearances are listed in Table 3.

Table 3: Characteristic postmortem observations in fatal morphine poisoning

External	*Internal*
Injection marks. Deep cyanosis of face and nails	Characteristic odor of opium in stomach
Intense, marked lividity (turns black after death)	Froth in airways. Pulmonary edema
Froth at mouth and nostrils	Organs are congested

Diagnosis

Marquis's test

A mixture of 3 mL concentrated H_2SO_4 and 3 drops of formalin is added to the sample to be analyzed. Color changes to purple followed by black, if positive.

Medicolegal significance or circumstances of poisoning

The medicolegal significance or circumstances of poisoning are described as follows:

- *Suicides:* Opium is often considered as ideal suicidal poison as the death is painless.
- *Homicides:* Rare due to its bitter taste and characteristic odor. Its misuse in infanticide remains a possibility.
- *Euthanasia:* Morphine is one of the preferred drug in euthanasia.
- *Accidental deaths:* It may occur due to therapeutic overdose, overdose in addicts or drugging of children to make them sleep.
- *Opium addiction:* Opium is mostly taken orally. Some of the peculiar ways of opium intake are: *Kasoomba* (poppy tea: decoction made from boiling opium poppies), *Halwa* (juice of unripe poppy capsules) and *Chandu or Madak* (smoking of opium).
- *Drug traffickers or body packers and body packer syndrome:* "Body packers" are individuals smuggling illicit drugs (heroin, cocaine, etc.) in their bodies across international borders. Intoxication due to the rupture of packets or condoms containing drugs in the gastrointestinal tract (GIT) is called "body packer syndrome" (For details, *see Chapter 19 on Drug Dependence and Drug Abuse*).
- Other significant facts regarding opium:
  - Licenses are issued for cultivation of poppy plant in India. Cultivation is under strict Government supervision in accordance with the Narcotic Drugs and Psychotropic Substances (NDPS) Act, 1985, and for pharmaceutical purposes only. Opium in India is grown in Rajasthan, Madhya Pradesh and Uttar Pradesh (***Golden Quadrangle:*** Varanasi, Lucknow, Bareilly, Badauin).
  - *Opium Wars:* These were fought for favored trade practices and legalization of the opium trade in China. The First Opium War (1839–1842) was fought between the British and the Chinese and the Second Opium War (1856–1860) or the "Arrow War" fought by the British and French against the Chinese.
  - *Illicit opium:* Two key regions of opium production and its illicit trafficking are referred as:
    - ◊ ***Golden Crescent:*** It includes Pakistan, Afghanistan and Iran. Afghanistan is the single largest producer of opium. Golden crescent also leads in *Cannabis* production.

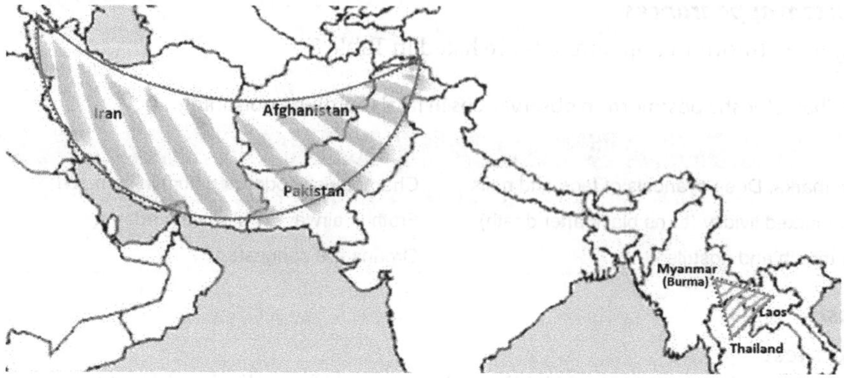

Fig. 1: Illicit trafficking of opium across the Golden Crescent and Golden Triangle areas.

◊ ***Golden Triangle:*** It includes opium producing areas of Myanmar (Burma), Laos and Thailand (North), which produces nearly 1/4th of world's opium (Fig. 1).

Write a note on chronic morphine poisoning?

Chronic morphine poisoning/morphinism/morphinomania/opium addiction

Opium is a highly addictive product. Opium addicts can tolerate 3–6 grams of opium per day. Long-term use of morphine causes psychological and physical dependence and tolerance.

Clinical manifestations

Anorexia, nausea, dry furred tongue, constipation, emaciation, weakness, constricted pupils, irritability, insomnia, impotence, moral and mental deterioration, dementia and hallucinations. Pigmentation and scarring is associated with repeated injections, and addicts often resort to tattooing to conceal it.

Management

- Drug (morphine) should be withdrawn gradually. Abrupt stoppage causes withdrawal symptoms
- *Methadone* (oral) is the *drug of choice* (dose of methadone is tapered and gradually withdrawn)
- *Withdrawal symptoms:* It appears 6–8 hours after stopping the drug, known as **"cold turkey"**. Symptoms include sweating, yawning, lacrimation, sneezing, rhinorrhea, anxiety, restlessness, *dilated pupils, diarrhea,* dehydration, muscle spasms and weight loss, etc.
- Withdrawal symptoms are treated with *methadone* (oral).

Write a short note on Heroin addiction?

- *Heroin (diacetylmorphine)* also called *brown sugar, smack, junk, dope,* etc. is a synthetic derivative of opium. Heroin is more than 2 times as potent as morphine
- Heroin has a strong narcotic analgesic effect; its euphoric effect is primarily due to its metabolites

- Heroin is rapidly metabolized, and hence, cannot be detected in blood after half to 1 hour of intravenous (IV) administration. It may, however, be detected in urine for a much longer time

Heroin → 6-monoacetylmorphine (a highly potent μ receptor agonist) → Morphine (detected in chemical analysis)

- Heroin can be smoked, snuffed or injected. Tolerance occurs rapidly in heroin addicts
- Popular forms of heroin among addicts are *brown sugar and black tar (Mexican heroin).*

Clinical manifestations

- Anorexia, constipation, emaciation, weakness, impotence, moral and mental deterioration, etc.
- Repeated injections cause pigmentation and scarring of the injection site. IV administration (mainlining) is associated with **"needle track ulcers"**, while intramuscular (IM) or subcutaneous (SC) injections (skin popping) are associated with map shaped **"geographical ulcers"**
- Drug abuser's elbow (myositis ossificans), heroin associated nephropathy and endocarditis are other complications
- Use or sharing of non-sterile needles can cause local abscesses, systemic infections such as human immunodeficiency virus (HIV), hepatitis, etc. and enlarged regional lymph nodes.

CHAPTER 11

Neurotoxics: Inebriants

Enlist the commercial preparations of alcohol (Ethyl alcohol/Ethanol/C_2H_5OH). Mention some common alcoholic beverages. Write a note on Proof spirit?

The commercial preparations of alcohol (ethyl alcohol/ethanol/C_2H_5OH) are listed in Table 1.

Table 1: Commercial preparations of ethyl alcohol

Preparation	Constituents
Absolute alcohol (anhydrous alcohol, dehydrated alcohol)	99.5% ethanol (range between 99% and 100%)
Rectified spirit (rectified alcohol, neutral spirit)	95% ethanol
Methylated spirit (denatured alcohol)	90% ethanol, 9.5% methanol, 0.5% pyridine
Surgical spirit	95% ethanol, 5% methanol with oil of wintergreen

Common alcoholic beverages and their alcohol content are shown in Table 2.

Table 2: Common alcoholic beverages and their alcohol content

Beverages	Alcohol content (v/v)
Beer	4–8%
Champagne, wine	7–15% (14–24% in fortified wines)
Brandy, gin, vodka, whisky, rum	40–50% (may be as high as 75–95%)

Proof spirit

- Proof spirit is used to express concentration of alcohol in alcoholic beverages
- It refers to that concentration of ethanol which weighs exactly 12/13 of the weight of an equal volume of distilled water at 11°C. Proof strength is expressed in degrees
- 100 proof (UK) = 57.06% ethanol by volume, or 48.24% ethanol by weight
- Spirits weaker than 57.06% are called "underproof" while those stronger are referred as "overproof"
- Now, alcohol proof as a measure of alcohol content is replaced by alcohol by volume (ABV)
- Alcohol proof (USA) = Twice the percentage of ABV or 2.5 times alcohol by weight.

Write a note on the toxicokinetics (absorption, metabolism, distribution and excretion) of alcohol or ethanol?

Absorption

About 20% of alcohol is absorbed from the stomach and 80% from the small intestine. Absorption of ethanol is rapid, and maximum blood alcohol concentration (BAC) is reached in 45-90 minutes of alcohol intake.

Factors modifying the rate of absorption of alcohol are illustrated in Table 3.

Table 3: Factors modifying the rate of absorption

Absorption is increased or faster in	*Absorption is slower or delayed in*
Hard drinks (higher alcohol concentration)	Beer, wine, etc. (lower alcohol concentration)
Warm drinks (due to capillary dilatation)	Cooled drinks
Drinks taken empty stomach	Intake with food (delayed gastric emptying)
Diluted alcohol (taken with water, etc.)	Concentrated alcohol (neat drink)
Drinks taken with carbonated drinks (due to increased surface area of bubbles)	Drinks taken with water or juices when compared to carbonated drinks
Individuals after gastrectomy	Achlorhydria and in chronic gastritis

Note
- Absorption of alcohol is delayed in concentrated drinks due to gastric mucosal irritation and pyloric spasm
- Mixing of drinks cause increased gastric emptying and thus increased absorption from intestines.

Metabolism

Metabolism of alcohol takes place in the liver through:
- Alcohol dehydrogenase pathway (oxidation involving two steps as described below)
- Microsomal ethanol oxidizing system
- Peroxidase catalase system.

The majority of the alcohol is metabolized in the liver by alcohol dehydrogenase pathway:

$$\text{Ethanol} \xrightarrow{\substack{\text{Alcohol}\\ \text{dehydrogenase}}} \text{Acetaldehyde} \xrightarrow{\substack{\text{Aldehyde}\\ \text{dehydrogenase}}} \text{Acetic acid} \xrightarrow{\substack{\text{Krebs}\\ \text{cycle}}} CO_2 + H_2O$$

Ethanol is oxidized to acetaldehyde first and then to acetic acid by enzyme dehydrogenases, where *nicotinamide adenine dinucleotide* (NAD) acts as a coenzyme. Acetate then enters into the Krebs cycle to form carbon dioxide (CO_2) and water (H_2O).

Deranged liver functions → Decreased rate of metabolism → Prolonged intoxication

Distribution

Alcohol is distributed to all body tissues proportional to their water content. Most tissues and organs have high water content (70–80% water by weight), while adipose tissue and bone have low (10–20%) water content.

Note: Relative to weight, the aqueous compartment is smaller in females and obese individuals due to higher body fat content. Hence, for equal amounts of alcohol consumed by individuals of same weight, the BAC will be higher in females (approximately 25% more than males) and in obese individuals.

Relative alcohol concentration in viscera and body fluids at equilibrium* are shown in Table 4.

Table 4: Relative alcohol concentration in blood and viscera or body fluids at equilibrium*

Alcohol concentration	Relation
Arterial: Venous blood	1:1
Blood: Plasma or serum	1:1.12 to 1.2
Blood: Urine#	1:1.3
Blood: Liver or brain	1:0.85
Blood: Alveolar air	2100:1

*Relative alcohol concentration varies in the absorption phase before the equilibrium is established. In absorption phase venous BAC is approximately 10% lesser than arterial BAC.
#Urinalysis is highly unreliable in estimation of BAC.

Elimination and excretion

Elimination of alcohol occurs by its metabolism and excretion. 90% of the alcohol is metabolized (oxidized) in liver and only 10% is excreted as such from the body (5% in urine and 5% through the breath). Insignificant amounts are also excreted in sweat, saliva and milk.

Alcohol follows zero order elimination kinetics (rate of elimination is independent of its concentration). The rate of fall of BAC is 10–20 mg% per hour.

Note: *Blood alcohol concentration (BAC) or blood alcohol level (BAL):* It is the quantification (quantity) of alcohol in the body. Approximately 5% of the alcohol is excreted unchanged through the breath that forms the basis of breath alcohol testing to estimate the BAC at the time of the test.

Write a note on acute alcohol or ethanol intoxication and its management? Mention the specific postmortem findings in deaths due to alcohol intoxication?

Mechanism of toxicity or action

- Alcohol crosses the blood-brain barrier and cause central nervous system (CNS) depressant effects
- *Frontal lobe depression:* Cause mood changes, lack of judgment
- *Occipital lobe depression:* Cause visual disturbances
- *Cerebellar depression:* Cause motor incoordination, decreased reaction time
- *Reticular activating system depression:* Results in loss of consciousness
- *Brain stem depression:* Cardiovascular and/or respiratory depression (cause of death).
- Alcohol also has a direct depressant action on the heart

Clinical manifestations of acute alcohol intoxication

Clinical manifestations of acute alcohol intoxication are shown in Table 5. Other associated effects of alcohol intoxication include:

Alcoholic blackout: It refers to acute anterograde amnesia (without loss of consciousness) after rapid consumption of moderate to large amounts of alcohol. Blackouts in chronic alcohol ingestion, are often referred to as the "alcoholic palimpsest".

Micturition syncope (fainting during urination): Alcohol or heavy beer drinking may trigger this condition (alcohol-induced postural hypotension). The loss of consciousness is transient.

Table 5: Clinical manifestations of acute alcohol intoxication

BAC (mg%)		Stage	Manifestations
<50		Sobriety *(decent)*	None or apparently normal
50–100	State of Excitement	Euphoria *(delighted and devilish)*	Feeling of well-being, overconfidence, talkativeness, lack of inhibitions, mood swings, decreased attention, *dilated pupils, alcohol gaze nystagmus (HGN)*[*]
100–150		Excitement *(delirious)*	Mild muscular incoordination, increased reaction time, lack of self-control and judgment, poor concentration, mildly slurred speech
150–200	State of incoordination	Confusion *(dazed)*	Confusion, disorientation, muscular incoordination, slurred speech, staggering gait, visual disturbances (diplopia and dilated pupils), flushed face, drowsiness, decreased response to stimuli, vomiting
200–300		Stupor *(dejected)*	
300–500	State of coma	Coma *(dead drunk)*	Loss of consciousness, diminished or loss of reflexes, labored breathing, subnormal temperature, rapid pulse, *constricted pupils, positive Macewen's sign*[#]
>500		Death *(dead)*	Respiratory failure *(cause of death)*

[*]*Alcohol gaze nystagmus:* It is the involuntary, jerky movement of the eye due to the effects of alcohol on the vestibulo-ocular system. It can be horizontal gaze nystagmus (HGN) in the direction of the gaze when the head is still in sitting or standing position and positional alcohol nystagmus (PAN) on turning the head in supine position.

[#]*Macewen's sign:* Pupils are constricted in alcoholic coma (BAC >300 mg%). Macewen's sign refers to the transient dilatation of already constricted pupils on applying any mechanical stimuli (pinching the skin/slapping/pressing the sternal area with knuckle).

Abbreviations: BAC, blood alcohol concentration; HGN, horizontal gaze nystagmus

Hangover (after-effect): Heavy drinking in night is frequently followed by nausea, fatigue, headache, body ache, irritability, etc. on the next morning. Dehydration and hypoglycemia are the likely causes for hangovers.

Fatal dose

150–250 mL of absolute alcohol taken in 1 hour. *BAC more than 500 mg% is lethal.*

Fatal period

12–24 hours.

Management

- Maintain airway, breathing and circulation
- Gastric lavage, preferably with an alkaline solution
- Prevention from aspiration (keep the patient in left lateral position, and keep airways clear)
- *Intravenous fluids:* 1 liter normal saline, 10% glucose, 15 units of insulin and 100 mg thiamine
- Hemodialysis or peritoneal dialysis when BAC is very high and liver functions are impaired.

Postmortem appearances

The major postmortem findings are listed as follows:

- *External:* Congested conjunctiva
- *Internal:* Alcoholic odor in stomach and cavities. Organs are congested. Signs of aspiration may be seen.

- *Specimens for Regional Forensic Science Laboratory:* Routine viscera, blood from the peripheral veins (femoral preferably), vitreous, urine, brain, cerebrospinal fluid (CSF), lungs, epidural hematoma (EDH) or subdural hematoma (SDH). Subdural clot gives an accurate estimate of the alcohol concentration at the time of head injury.

Write a note on chronic alcohol abuse/chronic alcoholism/alcohol addiction and its management?

Chronic alcoholics or alcohol addicts are individuals who cannot stay away from alcohol for long, and experience withdrawal symptoms on any attempt to stop drinking. Dependence is both physical and psychological. Tolerance develops gradually and the alcohol addicts need to take relatively higher quantities of alcohol to get the same effect.

Five subtypes of chronic alcoholism are described in the Table 6.

Table 6: Subtypes of chronic alcoholism

Subtypes	*Dependence*	*Features*
Alpha alcoholism	Psychological dependence only	Normal body functions
Beta alcoholism	No physical dependence	Physical disease states in alcoholism
Gamma alcoholism	Mild physical dependence	Tolerance, withdrawal symptoms
Delta alcoholism	Strong physical dependence	Tolerance, withdrawal symptoms
Epsilon alcoholism	Periodic binges, dipsomania	Paroxysmal or periodic alcoholism

Chronic alcoholism is often associated with the following:

- *Tolerance and dependence* (Tolerance develops primarily due to CNS adaptation, and also increased rate of alcohol metabolism due to larger amounts of enzymes produced by liver). In liver damage, *reverse tolerance* occurs and lesser amounts produce higher intoxication.
- *Alcoholic hepatitis and cirrhosis* (Most common complication, leading to liver failure)
- *Chronic gastritis, peptic ulceration* (May cause absorption defects)
- *Mallory-Weiss syndrome* (Lower esophageal mucosal tear and hemorrhage)
- *Chronic pancreatitis* (Dose-dependent effect of alcohol abuse)
- *Peripheral neuropathy* (Most common neurological abnormality. Effects include *allodynia*, weakness, unsteady gait, wrist and foot drop)
- *Alcoholic hallucinosis* (Persistent auditory or visual hallucinations within 48 hours of intake)
- *Thiamine (vitamin B_1) deficiency* [*Wernicke's encephalopathy (WE), Korsakoff's psychosis (KP)*]
- *Alcoholic cardiomyopathies: Myocarditis* due to toxic effects of alcohol and its metabolites, *Munich beer heart* (cardiac dilatation and hypertrophy in heavy beer drinkers)
- *Other cardiac conditions* (*Beriberi heart* due to thiamine deficiency, *Dysrhythmias*)
- *Endocrine and metabolic disorders* (Gynecomastia, testicular atrophy, thyroid disorders)
- *Alcohol amblyopia or nutritional optic neuropathy* (Painless and gradual loss of vision)
- *Fetal alcohol syndrome* (Teratogenic effects due to alcohol abuse during pregnancy include mental retardation, microcephaly, facial abnormalities and growth deficiencies of the new born)
- *Marchiafava-Bignami syndrome* (Degeneration of corpus callosum—Dementia).

Mnemonic: A B C D E F G H–M4 (for easy recall of conditions associated with chronic alcoholism)			
A	Alcohol amblyopia	*E*	Encephalopathy, Endocrine disorders
B	B_1 deficiency (WKS)[#]	*F*	Fetal alcohol syndrome
C	Cirrhosis, Cardiomyopathies	*G*	Gastritis, Gynecomastia
D	Dysrhythmias, Dependence	*H*	Hepatitis, Hallucinosis
M4	Myocarditis, Munich beer heart, Mallory-Weiss syndrome, Marchiafava-Bignami syndrome		

[#] *Wernicke-Korsakoff syndrome:* It is due to thiamine deficiency in alcohol abuse.

Wernicke-Korsakoff syndrome (WKS) comprises of Wernicke's encephalopathy (WE) and Korsakoff's psychosis (KP) that usually coexist.

Wernicke's encephalopathy: It is a neurological disorder, and a medical emergency.

- Cause: Acute Vitamin B1 (thiamine) deficiency
- Lesions: Lesions in mammillary bodies, thalamic nuclei, hippocampi, pontomedullary tegmentum
- Clinical features: Classic triad of ataxia, encephalopathy and ophthalmoplegia, along with confusion, altered consciousness, delirium, disorientation and memory disturbances
- Treatment: Intravenous (IV) thiamine (50–100 mg), IV glucose.

Korsakoff's psychosis: A late neurological sequelae of Wernicke's encephalopathy.

- *Cause:* Vitamin B1 (thiamine) deficiency
- *Clinical features (**Mnemonic ACP or CAP**): **Amnesia*** (anterograde amnesia; inability to form new memories and retrograde amnesia; loss of memory or inability to recall information), *Confabulation* (filling up of memory gaps with imaginary events or ideas) and ***Polyneuropathy***
- *Treatment:* Intravenous thiamine, correction of electrolyte imbalance.

Management of chronic alcoholism

It comprises of medicinal therapy, conditional reflex therapy and psychotherapy.

Medicinal therapy

- Disulfiram (aldehyde dehydrogenase inhibitor)

Ethanol —(*Alcohol Dehydrogenase*)→ *Acetaldehyde* —(*Aldehyde Dehydrogenase*, crossed out)→ *Acetic acid*

Action: Aldehyde dehydrogenase inhibition cause accumulation of acetaldehyde resulting in unpleasant effects: *Aldehyde syndrome*

Aldehyde syndrome (alcohol flush reaction) is characterized by nausea, flushing, palpitation, headache, tightness of chest, sweating, abdominal cramps, hypotension, etc. Alcoholic develops an aversion to alcohol due to the above mentioned unpleasant symptoms.

Dose of disulfiram (antabuse): 250 mg OD orally (dose is tapered gradually over months).

Contraindications of disulfiram therapy: Hepatotoxicity, nephrotoxicity and pregnancy.

Note: Alcohol flush reaction can be seen after alcohol consumption in individuals with inherited deficiency of enzyme aldehyde dehydrogenase due to accumulation of acetaldehyde.

- *Citrated calcium carbimide:* 50 mg OD (action is similar to disulfiram)
- *N-methyl-D-aspartate (NMDA) receptor blockers (acamprosate, memantine):* It is useful in alcohol dependence
- *Ondansetron (5-HT3 serotonin receptor antagonist):* It reduces craving for alcohol
- *Naltrexone (opioid receptor antagonist):* It reduces craving for alcohol
- *Vitamin supplements:* Thiamine
- *Others:* Benzodiazepines, chlorpromazine, clonidine, etc.

Conditioned reflex therapy

Various alcoholic drinks are given together with drugs that cause nausea and vomiting for a week. Later on mere sight of the bottles causes unpleasant symptoms, and thus, an aversion towards alcohol.

Supportive psychotherapy

It includes individual therapy and group therapy.

Alcoholic anonymous

It is an international mutual help group founded in 1935, and has branches all over the world. The primary purpose of the group is to help alcoholics stay away from alcohol. Members share their experiences with others through meetings, letters, etc. to solve their common problem and help each other to abstain from alcohol. Similar other groups exist today globally.

Write a short note on alcohol withdrawal syndrome (AWS) or Abstinence syndrome?

Alcohol withdrawal syndrome (AWS) comprises of symptoms seen in alcohol addicts on sudden discontinuance or stoppage of alcohol. In general, the symptoms include nausea, vomiting, diarrhea, tremors of the hands and tongue, restlessness, insomnia, fever, hallucinations, seizures, and delirium tremens, etc. The symptoms of AWS are described according to the severity and time elapsed after withdrawal in Table 7. The most serious of these is *Delirium tremens.*

Table 7: Symptoms of alcohol withdrawal syndrome according to the severity and time elapsed after withdrawal

Common abstinence syndrome	*Alcohol hallucinations*	*Seizures (rum fits)*	*Delirium tremens*
In 6–8 hours after stopping	In 24–36 hours	In about 48 hours	In 3–5 days
Nausea, headache, irritability, insomnia, tremors, anxiety	Auditory and visual hallucinations	Clonic-tonic type, unconsciousness	Fever, confusion, hallucinations, death
Mnemonic: ***WITHDRAW*** (**W**ithdrawal, **I**nsomnia, **T**remors, **T**achycardia, **H**allucinations, **H**ypertension, **D**iaphoresis, **D**elirium tremens, **D**elusion, **R**um fits, **A**nxiety, **A**gitation, **W**ithdrawal)			

Delirium tremens (DTs, the shakes, the horrors): It is an acute episode of delirium.

- *Precipitating factors:* Sudden alcohol withdrawal, trauma, acute infection
- *Onset:* 3–5 days after the sudden withdrawal of alcohol
- *Symptoms:* Agitation, confusion, disorientation, fever, sweating, hypertension or fluctuating blood pressure (BP), delusions, horrific hallucinations and even death may occur.

- Treatment:
  - Diazepam 5–10 mg IV (drug of choice) or lorazepam in deranged liver functions
  - Thiamine 50–100 mg, and correction of fluid and electrolyte imbalance.

Define drunkenness and alcohol intoxication. Describe the specific tests conducted to evaluate if an individual is intoxicated or not, and the format of final opinion furnished in these cases.

Drunkenness

In 1925, a special committee of the British Medical Association defined drunkenness as *"That the person concerned was so much under the influence of alcohol as to have lost control to such an extent as to render him unable to execute safely the occupation on which he was engaged at the material time".*

Drunkenness is often defined as *"a condition produced in a person who has taken alcohol in a quantity sufficient to cause him to lose control of his faculties to such an extent, that he is unable to execute safely the occupation on which he is engaged at the material time".*

The term "drunkenness" describes the behavior displayed by an individual who has consumed alcohol while in medicolegal context, "intoxication" is used to describe the effects of alcohol. The World Health Organization (WHO) defines acute intoxication as *"Intoxication is a condition that follows the administration of a psychoactive substance and results in disturbances in the level of consciousness, cognition, perception, judgment, affect, or behavior, or other psychophysiological functions and responses".*

Tests for drunkenness

Clinical examination taken up to evaluate if an individual is intoxicated or not is detailed in Table 8.

Table 8: Clinical examination to evaluate if an individual is intoxicated or not

Function	*Test and its description*	*Observations and inferences*
Speech	Test phrases or tongue twisters (e.g. Rashtrapati). Articulation and content is noted. Observe if there is blurring of certain consonants *It is one of the earliest sign of muscle incoordination.*	Slurred, thick or overprecise speech is suggestive of inebriation
Memory	Asking questions to find the ability to recall recent events, e.g. simple calculations, number of drinks taken, payments made, etc.	Alcohol blackout, retrograde amnesia is suggestive of inebriation
Orientation or alertness	Enquire about the time, day of the week, present location, etc.	Alertness effected at blood alcohol concentration (BAC) >100–150 mg%
Gait	**Walk-and-Turn (WAT) test:* Assess neuromuscular coordination by manner of walking, reaction time and manner of turning	Normal or staggering gait is suggestive of inebriation
Stance or balance	*Romberg's test (for cerebellar disturbances):* The person is asked to stand erect with his feet together and eyes closed	Test is positive if he sways or falls, suggestive of inebriation

Contd...

Contd...

Function	Test and its description	Observations and inferences
	[*] *One-leg stand (OLS) test:* The person is asked to stand with one foot off the ground for 30 seconds	Swaying, hopping, or using arms for support denotes positive test
Writing	The patient is asked to write or copy a phrase. Observe if he is able to write in a straight line, missing words and time taken for writing. Signature can be compared with those on identity cards	Disturbed strokes, distorted writings or signature are suggestive of inebriation
Neuromuscular coordination[#]	• *Finger nose test, finger-to-finger test:* The person is asked to close his or her eyes, and touch their nose with the tip of index finger • *Picking up pencil or coin from floor* • *Buttoning or unbuttoning the shirt*	• Under or overshooting is suggestive of inebriation • Nonperformance or inadequate performance is suggestive of inebriation
Reflexes	• Knee and ankle reflex • Plantar reflex (Babinski's sign)	• Delayed or sluggish • Extensor plantar response
Eyes	• *Conjunctiva:* Congestion due to peripheral vasodilation • *Pupillary reflex:* Check pupillary reaction time, repeat for 4–5 times • *Convergence:* Ask the patient to follow your finger-tip moving it in all directions, ask to converge gaze	• Congested • Sluggish, unequal pupil • Difficulty in smooth tracking or convergence
	[*] *Horizontal gaze nystagmus (HGN) or pen test:* Ask the patient to follow your finger or a pen moving it in horizontal axis till the peripheral fields on either side. Head is still in sitting or erect posture *Positional alcohol nystagmus (PAN):* Turning the head in supine position	Exaggerated, involuntary jerking movements of the eye that occurs at lower angles (within 45° of center) is suggestive of inebriation
	Macewen's sign: Pinching the skin/slapping/pressing the sternal area with knuckle	Transient dilation of the already constricted pupils in alcoholic coma (BAC >300 mg%)

[*] *WAT, OLS and HGN* are the three tests included in *Standardized Field Sobriety Test (SFST)* employed by the police officers in the United States of America (USA) to determine if a driver is impaired due to alcohol consumption.
[#] Before assessing the neuromuscular integrity, presence of any CNS diseases should be ruled out.

The final opinion based on clinical examination is marked as one of the 3 choices given below.

Opinion

Based on the clinical examination, I am of the opinion that Mr. or Ms........:

- Has not consumed alcohol
- Has consumed alcohol but, is not under its influence
- Has consumed alcohol and is under its influence.

Blood or urine samples are preserved and sent for chemical analysis to determine the concentration of alcohol at the Regional Forensic Science Laboratory (RFSL).

Note: The final diagnosis of alcohol intoxication should be based on toxicological evidence. Blood or urine is preserved in sodium fluoride and analyzed to estimate concentration of alcohol.

Widmark's formula

It is used to estimate the alcohol concentration in the body.

The formula applied for blood is $a = cpr$ and for urine the formula is $a = 3/4\ qpr$.

- *a:* Quantity of alcohol consumed (grams)
- *c:* Concentration of alcohol in blood (gram/liter or decigrams%)
- *p:* Body weight (kilograms)
- *r:* Constant (0.68 in men; 0.55 in women)
- *q:* Concentration of alcohol in urine (gram/liter or decigrams%).

Describe the various issues associated with alcohol consumption and drunkenness. Mention the medicolegal aspects or circumstances of acute alcohol intoxication?

Medicolegal significance and circumstances of acute alcohol intoxication

The circumstances of acute alcohol intoxication are described as follows:

- *Alcohol in violence and criminal behavior:* Alcohol is commonly implicated in a vast number of homicides, domestic violence cases, sexual assaults (alcohol-facilitated sexual assaults or rape), traffic accidents and suicides. Alcohol is the most common substance associated with "date rape" in India and worldwide

  A solution of chloral hydrate and alcohol referred to as "knockout drops" or "Mickey Finn" is notoriously implicated in drug facilitated sexual assaults or date rapes.
- *Drunken driving/alcohol, traffic accidents and the law:* Alcohol is one of the leading causes of road traffic accidents.
  - Rise in BAC progressively impairs driving ability due to the reasons as listed in Box 1.

Box 1: Effect of higher BAC on the driving ability	
• Increased reaction time • Over confidence (more risk taking behavior) • Loss of concentration • Impaired judgment ability	• Impaired muscular coordination • Fine movements affected most • Diminished peripheral vision and blurring • Impaired auditory acuity

  - The provisions of The Motor Vehicles Act (MVA), 1988 that are significant with regard to drunken driving are Section 185, 202, 203, 204 and 205 of MVA:
    - ◊ *Section 185 of the Motor Vehicles Act:* Driving by a drunken person or by a person under the influence of drugs is a punishable offence in India, if such individual has:
      - Blood alcohol *exceeding 30 mg/100 mL* of blood as detected by a breath analyzer test
      - *Punishment for the 1st offence:* Imprisonment up to 6 months or fine up to ₹ 2000 or both
      - *For another offence within 3 years:* Imprisonment up to 2 years or fine up to ₹ 3000 or both.
    - ◊ *Section 202 of the Motor Vehicles Act:* Police officer has the power to arrest a person without warrant in drunken driving. The accused must be produced for medical examination within 2 hours or else the accused has to be released from custody
    - ◊ *Section 203 of the Motor Vehicles Act:* It describes the procedures for breath tests. The findings of the breath test are admissible evidence in the court of law

◊ *Section 204 of the Motor Vehicles Act:* It describes the procedures for laboratory tests, i.e. analysis of blood at Government approved laboratories. The evidence is admissible in the court of law
◊ *Section 205 of the Motor Vehicles Act:* Refusal for a breath test is presumption of unfitness to drive.

Note: *Excessive drinking* refers to drinking beyond the permissible limits prescribed by the laws of the land. The permissible limit of BAC for driving in India is 30 mg%. In the neighboring countries of Nepal, Pakistan and Bangladesh it is 0 mg% (not permitted). The permissible limits of BAC in most other countries range between 50 mg% and 80 mg%.

- *Consent and drunkenness:* In general, no person should be examined or any samples preserved without their consent. However, consent is not mandatory for examination of an arrested person for drunkenness in accordance with Section 53 of the Criminal Procedure Code (CrPC)

  Note: In hospitalization following alleged acute alcohol intoxication, treat the case as medicolegal case (MLC) (see Chapter 4 for details on Medicolegal Duties of Doctor in an Alleged Case of Poisoning).

- *Criminal responsibility and alcohol:* These are set in interrelated Sections 85 and 86 of the Indian Penal Code (IPC).
  - *Section 85 Indian Penal Code: Nothing is an offence which is done by a person who, at the time of doing it, is, by reason of intoxication, incapable of knowing the nature of the act, or that he is doing what is either wrong, or contrary to law; provided that the thing which intoxicated him was administered to him without his knowledge or against his will*
  - *Section 86 Indian Penal Code:* Voluntary drunkenness cannot be pleaded as a defense for *offences requiring a particular intent or knowledge committed by one who is intoxicated.*
  - *Delirium tremens* is a disorder that is considered as a defense in criminal responsibility
  - *Mania a potu (pathological alcohol intoxication):* It is a rare condition where consumption of small quantities of alcohol causes violent behavior and subsequent amnesia for the behavior and actions caused. Criminals may plead it as a defense for the crime committed.
- *Alcohol and sudden death:* Alcohol induced arrhythmias are the cause of sudden deaths
- *Holiday heart syndrome:* Atrial fibrillation (AF) after an alcohol binge (binge refers to consumption of more than 4–5 drinks in 2 hours)
- *Alcohol and drug abuse:* Alcohol is the most common substance of abuse in India
- *Alcohol and medical practice/professional misconduct:* Practicing medicine after consuming alcohol is considered as infamous conduct
- *Alcoholic coma versus coma due to head injury:* General appearance, alcohol odor and Macewen's sign, etc. help to diagnose the cause of unconsciousness as alcohol intoxication
- *Civil responsibility and alcohol:* Contracts signed in inebriated state are invalid
- *Endogenous production of alcohol:* Alcohol production can occur in the body during life and after death.
  - *During life:* Due to bacterial activity in the gastrointestinal (GI) tract. Endogenous production of alcohol in individuals suffering from intestinal candidiasis is known as *auto-brewery syndrome*
  - *After death:* Alcohol production can occur due to the microbial activity during putrefaction
  - Collected blood samples if not sterile are prone to fermentation by bacteria, yeast or fungi causing alcohol production.

In all such cases alcohol estimates can be erroneous. Urine and vitreous resist putrefaction and hence, are preferred samples for alcohol estimation especially in putrefied bodies. Use of preservatives and refrigeration inhibits microbial activity and postmortem production of ethanol.

Describe the mechanism of toxicity, clinical manifestations, and management of methyl alcohol poisoning. Mention its medicolegal significance?

Methyl alcohol/methanol/wood alcohol/wood spirit/wood naphtha (CH_3OH)

Mechanism of action

Methyl alcohol is metabolized in the liver by alcohol dehydrogenase pathway:

$$\text{Methanol} \xrightarrow[\text{dehydrogenase}]{\text{Alcohol}} \text{Formaldehyde} \xrightarrow[\text{dehydrogenase}]{\text{Aldehyde}} \text{Formic acid} \xrightarrow[\text{metabolism}]{\text{Folate dependent}} CO_2 + H_2O$$

Methanol is oxidized to formaldehyde first and then to formic acid by enzyme dehydrogenases (similar to ethanol metabolism). Further metabolism of formic acid is slow and folate-dependent. The rate of oxidation of methanol, however, is slower (1/5th) than ethanol, and so its accumulation on repeat doses is reported. The metabolites of methanol, formaldehyde and formic acid (predominantly) are responsible for its toxic effects.

Clinical manifestations

The clinical manifestations are illustrated in Table 9.

Table 9: Clinical manifestations of methyl alcohol poisoning

System involved	*Clinical manifestations*
Gastrointestinal system	Nausea, vomiting, abdominal pain
Central nervous system	Headache, vertigo, neck stiffness, confusion. Parkinson-like extrapyramidal symptoms and coma in severe intoxication
Respiratory system	Dyspnea, cyanosis, odor of alcohol in breath
Cardiovascular system	Tachycardia, hypotension
Urinary or renal system	Metabolic acidosis, acute tubular necrosis, anuria
Ocular toxicity (Photoreceptors, Müller cells, and retrolaminar portion of the optic nerve are affected)	Dilated pupils, blurred vision, photophobia, painful eye movements, loss of pupillary reflex, disturbances of color vision, visual field defects, diminished visual acuity, *blindness* due to optic neuritis and atrophy in severe toxicity. *"Flickering white spots before the eyes" or "being in a snowstorm"* is characteristic of methanol intoxication

Specific toxicity: Ocular toxicity (retinal damage and blindness) and renal toxicity (metabolic acidosis) is caused due to metabolites of methanol; formaldehyde and formic acid.

Fatal dose

60–250 mL or blood methanol concentration more than 200 mg%.

Fatal period

24–36 hours.

Cause of death

Respiratory failure (most common), CNS depression, or renal failure.

Management

The management of methyl alcohol poisoning is described as follows:

- Shift the patient to quiet and dark room, and protect the eyes from light
- *Gastric lavage* with 5% sodium bicarbonate solution (500 mL may be left in the stomach)
- *Sodium bicarbonate* (oral or IV administration) for treatment of metabolic acidosis
- *Ethanol (specific antidote)* has *increased affinity to the enzyme alcohol dehydrogenase* (ADH), and causes competitive inhibition of the oxidation of methanol to its toxic metabolite formaldehyde as shown in Flowchart 1. Ethanol is administered by IV infusion (10% ethanol in a dose of 10 mL/kg, with serum level maintained at 100 mg%.) till the blood methanol levels fall below 25 mg%. Alternatively, 95% ethanol can be administered orally (1 mL/kg) in 200 mL fruit juice over 30 minutes, followed by a maintenance dose of 50% ethanol. Only issue is the inebriation caused in this therapy.
- *Fomepizole [4-methylpyrazole (4MP)], a specific ADH inhibitor* is considered as *the antidote of* choice. It prevents oxidation of methanol to its toxic metabolite formaldehyde as shown in Flowchart 1. The treatment is, however, not easily available and costly
- *Hemodialysis* is the mainstay in the treatment. It brings about early elimination of methanol and its metabolites, thus protecting the patient of the toxic effects and reducing the duration of antidotal therapy
- *Folinic acid or leucovorin (calcium folinate)* 1 mg/kg IV reduces the blood formate levels by increasing formic acid metabolism, thus protecting from effects of metabolic acidosis, etc. (Flowchart 1).
- *Symptomatic and supportive treatment* (e.g.; diazepam for treating seizures).

Flowchart 1: Specific treatment of methyl alcohol poisoning and the mechanism of action of its antidotes

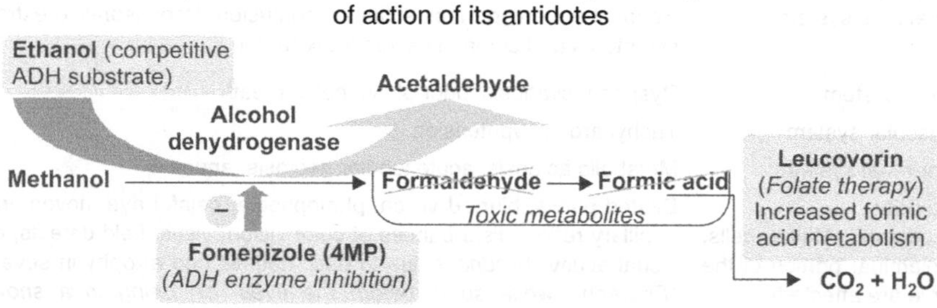

Abbreviation: ADH, alcohol dehydrogenase

Medicolegal significance and circumstances of methyl alcohol poisoning

The medicolegal significance and circumstances of methyl alcohol poisoning include:

- *Liquor tragedies or Hooch tragedies:* Consumption of illicit or spurious liquor adulterated with methanol has caused mass blindness and fatalities in many states of India and abroad
- Poisoning occurs following unintentional or intentional ingestion of products where methanol is present as a solvent (antifreeze, cleaning solutions, dyes, varnish, paint remover or thinner, etc.).

Note: Arrack is a distilled alcoholic drink made from either the fermented sap of coconut flowers, sugarcane, grains or fruit, etc. It is produced mainly in South Asia region (Arrack and illicit or spurious liquor are not the same entities).

Write a short note on ethylene glycol (EG) poisoning?

The metabolism and action of ethylene glycol, along with clinical manifestations and management of its poisoning are shown in Table 10.

Note: Oxalate crystals can be observed postmortem in various organs (liver, kidney, etc.).

Table 10: Metabolism and action of ethylene glycol, along with clinical manifestations and management of its poisoning

Metabolism and action of ethylene glycol

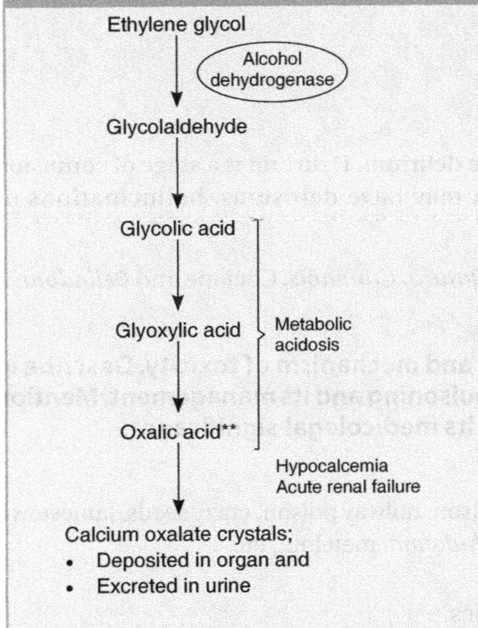

Clinical manifestations of acute poisoning:
1st stage (central nervous system depression) up to 12 hours: Nausea, vomiting, inebriation, confusion, convulsions, coma
2nd stage (cardiopulmonary dysfunction) in 12–24 hours: Tachycardia, tachypnea, hypotension, circulatory failure
3rd stage (renal dysfunction) in 24–72 hours: Metabolic acidosis (due to accumulation of glycolic and oxalic acid), oliguria, acute renal failure, hypocalcemia (oxalate binds with serum calcium to form calcium oxalate crystals that are deposited in organs and excreted in urine)
Management: (very similar to methanol poisoning)
Fomepizole and ethanol are specific antidotes. These inhibit enzyme alcohol dehydrogenase (ADH) and prevent the metabolism of ethylene glycol to toxic metabolites
Intravenous sodium bicarbonate to treat metabolic acidosis
Hemodialysis
10% calcium gluconate (calcium salts) is administered in severe hypocalcemia
Symptomatic treatment (mechanical ventilation, diazepam, etc.)

Note: Oxalate crystals can be observed in various organs (liver, kidney, etc.) at autopsy.

**For details on action and manifestations of oxalic acid poisoning see Chapter 5 on Corrosives.

CHAPTER 12

Neurotoxics: Deliriants

The deliriant poisons act on the brain and cause delirium. Delirium is a stage of confusion with altered sense of consciousness. Person may have delusions, hallucinations or excitement.

Deliriants: Some of the common deliriants are *Datura*, *Cannabis*, Cocaine and *Belladonna*, etc.

Write a note on Datura, its active principles and mechanism of toxicity. Describe in detail the clinical manifestations of Datura poisoning and its management. Mention the circumstances of Datura poisoning, i.e. its medicolegal significance.

Datura

It is also known popularly as thorn apple, road poison, railway poison, crazy seeds, Jamestown or Jimsonweed, devil's apple, devil's trumpet, *Belladonna*, metelnut, etc.

The two common species of the plant are:

1. *Datura stramonium:* It is found in high altitudes.
2. *Datura fastuosa:* It is found in plains. Two of its varieties are:
   - *Datura alba:* It has white flowers
   - *Datura niger:* It has dark purple or dark flowers.

Active principles

All parts of the plant are poisonous but the seeds and flowers are more toxic. The active principles (alkaloids) present in the plant are:

- Hyoscine (scopolamine)
- Hyoscyamine
- Traces of atropine.

Mechanism of toxicity

The alkaloids competitively block the neurotransmitter acetylcholine at muscarinic receptor, centrally and peripherally, and also at end-organ sites of parasympathetic nervous system. The stage of overstimulation of the nervous system is followed by the stage of depression. Scopolamine crosses blood-brain barrier and is responsible for the central nervous system (CNS) effects like delirium, drowsiness, agitation and dementia.

Clinical manifestations

Apart from vomiting and pain abdomen, the signs and symptoms are easily described as ***12 Ds of Datura poisoning:***

- **Dryness of mouth and throat, intense feeling of thirst**
- **Difficulty in talking, slurred speech**
- **Dysphagia, difficulty in swallowing**
- **Dilatation of pupils with loss of accommodation for near vision**
- **Diplopia, photophobia**
- **Dry hot skin, with flushing, hyperpyrexia, dilatation of cutaneous blood vessels**
- **Dysuria, urinary retention, bladder distention**
- **Drunken gait (ataxia), hyperreflexia**
- **Delirium (muttering) with visual or auditory hallucinations, agitation, amnesia, incoherence**
- **Delusions**
- **Drowsiness leading to convulsions, coma**
- **Death due to respiratory depression or failure.**

The manifestations are described in classic *Morton Still's* phrase:

Red as a beet (Flushing), ***blind as a bat*** (Diplopia, dilated pupils), ***hot as a hare*** (Hyperpyrexia), ***dry as a bone*** (Decreased secretions), ***mad as a hatter*** (Delirium).

Characteristic features of datura intoxication

- *Muttering delirium:* The delirious victim is silent or mutters indistinct and inaudible words
- *Carphologia and pill rolling:* Delirious victim makes some purposeless movements like pulling imaginary threads (*carphologia*), threading imaginary needle (*pill rolling*).

Note: Carphologia refers to picking or grasping of imaginary objects often seen in delirious or semiconscious patients.

Cause of death

Respiratory failure or cardiac arrhythmias.

Fatal dose

50–100 seeds (stupefying dose: 40–50 seeds).

Treatment

- *Gastrointestinal decontamination:* Gastric lavage
- *Physiological antidote: Physostigmine* crosses blood-brain barrier so is preferred over neostigmine, pyridostigmine, or pilocarpine. Use of physostigmine itself is debatable as it makes the patient vulnerable to hypotension, bradycardia convulsion and asystole
- Symptomatic and supportive treatment:
  - Tepid sponging for dry skin and to bring down the high temperature
  - Benzodiazepines to manage agitation
  - Artificial respiration, oxygen inhalation for patients with respiratory depression
  - Inhalation of bromide, short-acting barbiturates or ether for treating delirium.

Postmortem findings

Fragments of *Datura* seeds may be found in the stomach, even in the decomposed bodies as the seeds resist putrefaction for a long time. Otherwise the autopsy findings are nonspecific. (Visceral organs are congested.)

Medicolegal aspects and circumstances of datura poisoning

- Extract of the plant is mixed with eatables notably in the form of biscuits or in drinks and offered to unsuspecting passengers to rob them, or to individuals to commit kidnappings or sexual assaults. *Datura* for this reason is referred to as "road-side poison" or "railway poison"
- *Datura* is used to potentiate the effect of alcohol
- *Datura* is used in majun, and smoked with marijuana
- Scopolamine is used as "truth serum" during crime investigations or interrogations
- Accidental poisoning occurs when the *Datura* seeds are mistakenly consumed for capsicum seeds due to their close resemblance. Salient differences between the two are described in Table 1.
- *Datura* seeds resist putrefaction, and can be detected for long time after death.

Table 1: Differences between capsicum and datura seeds

Characteristics	*Capsicum (chilli) seeds*	*Datura seeds*
Size	Smaller	Larger
Color	Yellow	Brown
Shape	Round	Kidney shaped
Surface	Smooth	Pitted
Smell	Pungent	Odorless
Taste	Pungent	Bitter
Edges at convex border	Single	Double
Embryo on section	Curved inwards	Curved outwards

Note: See picture of *Datura* seeds and chilli seeds in Chapter 26 on Appliances and Spotters in Practical Examinations.

Write a note on Cannabis, its active principles and different preparations of Cannabis. Describe the clinical manifestations of acute and chronic cannabis poisoning and its management. Mention the circumstances of poisoning or its medicolegal significance.

Cannabis indica (Indian hemp, pot, weed, grass, rope, joint, reefer, Mary Jane, shit, etc.).

Active principles

Cannabinoids: Cannabinol, Cannabidiol; the active form is Δ9-tetrahydrocannabinol (THC).

Preparations of cannabis

Preparations of Cannabis in order of increasing potency include Bhang <Ganja <Hashish (Table 2). Other commonly used preparations of Cannabis are marijuana, majun, hash oil, sinsemilla, etc.

Table 2: Preparations of Cannabis with their potency and fatal doses

Preparation	*Common name*	*Source*	*THC*	*Fatal dose*
Bhang	Siddhi, sabji, patti	Dried leaves and shoots	10–15%	10 g/kg body weight
Ganja	Pot, weed, grass	Flowering tops of female plant	15–25%	8 g/kg body weight
Hashish	Charas (dried resin)	Leaves and stems	25–40%	2 g/kg body weight

Abbreviation: THC, Δ9-tetrahydrocannabinol

- *Marijuana or marihuana:* It is synonymous with *Cannabis* for its use as a psychoactive or therapeutic agent. It refers to dried leaves, flowers, stems, or seeds of *Cannabis* plant
  Marijuana is usually smoked in hand-rolled cigarettes (reefers or joints), emptied cigars filled with marijuana (packing the blunts), or in pipes or water pipes (bongs).
- *Majun/Majoon/Majoun:* Sweetmeat preparation of bhang/cannabis confections/dessert
- *Hash oil (hashish oil/honey oil/marijuana oil):* It is obtained by solvent extraction of *Cannabis*. It has a very high concentration of cannabinoids (THC)
- *Sinsemilla:* It is obtained from seedless female plant. It has high concentration of cannabinoids (THC).

Acute cannabis poisoning

The clinical manifestations of the two stages of acute *Cannabis* poisoning are described in Table 3.

Table 3: Clinical manifestations of acute Cannabis poisoning

I: Stage of excitement or euphoria	*II: Stage of narcosis or coma*
• Euphoria, sense of well-being, talkativeness, increased appetite and thirst, laughter or crying	• Tingling and numbness of extremities, giddiness, drowsiness, confusion
• Impaired memory, increased reaction time	• Motor incoordination, coma, collapse
• Visual hallucinations (usually sexual in nature)	• Respiratory depression

Note: Characteristic "burnt rope odor" is appreciable in the breath of those smoking Cannabis.

Management

- Secure airways and assisted respiration
- Gastric lavage and activated charcoal
- Anxiolytics (diazepam)
- Antipsychotics (haloperidol).

Cause of death

Respiratory failure.

Postmortem observations

Nonspecific. Organs are congested.

Medicolegal significance or circumstances of poisoning

- Recreational agent. Accidental poisoning may occur from its excessive intake
- May be used as stupefying agent to rob unsuspecting individuals.

Chronic cannabis poisoning

Prolonged intake of large quantities of *Cannabis* causes tolerance and some psychological dependence.

The manifestations of chronic *Cannabis* poisoning are:

- Anorexia, weight loss, muscle wasting, weakness, social withdrawal, moral and mental deterioration.
- Erectile dysfunction or impotence, and decreased sperm count, altered sperm size and shape thus, affecting fertility, decreased serum testosterone, gynecomastia, etc.

- Excessive use is characterized by CNS degeneration and insanity.
  - *Amotivational syndrome (rare):* It is characterized by apathy, dullness, lethargy and impaired judgment.
  - *Hashish insanity/charas insanity/hemp insanity:* It is characterized by mood swings, delusions (mostly delusion of persecution and delusion of grandeur), hallucinations (mostly visual and auditory) and amok.
  - *Run amok or running amok:* The person is possessed with murderous frenzy and goes on a killing spree. Such a person is highly aggressive, gets hold of any weapon and indiscriminately attacks anybody who comes in his or her way causing multiple fatalities. Subsequently in a stage of depression the person may surrender or commit suicide.

Management

Gradual withdrawal, sedatives, antipsychotics and psychotherapy.

Medicolegal significance and circumstances of poisoning

- Accidental deaths may occur due to its excessive intake
- No criminal responsibility in cases of run amok or for those suffering from hashish insanity [Section 84 Indian Penal Code (IPC)].

Write a note on Cocaine abuse?

Cocaine (coke, devil's dandruff, snow, white lady)

Cocaine is an alkaloid obtained from leaves of *Erythroxylum coca.*

It is usually snorted or sniffed, taken intravenously, or smoked as "crack".

(Crack is smokable form of cocaine obtained by mixing cocaine hydrochloride, baking soda and water).

Acute cocaine poisoning

Acute poisoning is characterized by stage of excitement followed by stage of depression.

Clinical manifestations include dilated pupils, hyperthermia, headache, seizures, tremors, tics, hypertension, arrhythmias, delirium, hallucinations, etc.

Lilliputian hallucinations or microptic hallucinations are often reported in acute poisoning.

Note: Lilliputian hallucinations are also reported in conditions such as delirium, schizophrenia, seizure disorders, and brain tumors.

Cause of death

Cardiac arrhythmias or myocardial infarction.

Medicolegal significance and circumstances of poisoning

Accidental deaths may occur due to cocaine overdose.

Chronic cocaine poisoning/cocainism/cocainomania/cocainophagia

Cocaine is a highly addictive drug, there is development of tolerance among addicts.

- Clinical manifestations of chronic poisoning include anorexia, emaciation, insomnia, anxiety, depression, psychosis, moral and mental deterioration.

- Intravenous cocaine abuse can cause local abscesses or culminates into endocarditis. Use or sharing of nonsterile needles can result in blood-borne infections such as human immunodeficiency virus (HIV), hepatitis, etc.
- Some of the characteristic manifestations of chronic cocaine poisoning include:
  - *Perforated nasal septum:* In cocaine snorting or sniffing. At times it results in flat saddle nose.
  - *Black teeth and tongue:* In cocaine abusers who rub cocaine to the gums.
  - *Crack eye:* It refers to corneal defects associated with exposure of eyes to cocaine smoke.
  - *Crack lung:* It refers to hemorrhagic alveolitis in cocaine abusers.
  - *Cocaine cardiomyopathies:* It is caused by cocaine induced damage to cardiac muscles.
  - *Cerebral atrophy:* It has been reported in cocaine abuse.
  - *Cocaine bug/coke bug/Magnan's symptoms/Magnan's phenomenon/Magnan-Saury's sign/formication/formicative hallucination/insect hallucination:* It refers to tactile hallucinations where an individual feels numerous ants or small insects crawling on or beneath the skin. The condition is associated with pruritus and excessive scratching.

Note: Crack baby refers to low-birth weight baby with congenital anomalies as a result of cocaine abuse during pregnancy.

Management

Gradual withdrawal and psychotherapy.

Cocaine withdrawal

Cocaine is often associated with only psychological and no physical dependence.

Cocaine withdrawal results in strong craving for the drug, fatigue, sleepiness, anxiety, irritability, agitation, restlessness, depression and suicidal tendencies.

Medicolegal significance and circumstances of poisoning

Drug traffickers/body packers/body packer syndrome: "Body packers" are individuals smuggling illicit drugs (heroin, cocaine, etc.) in their bodies across international borders. Rupture of packets or condoms containing drugs in the gastrointestinal tract (GIT) causes intoxication referred as "body packer syndrome" (For details, see Chapter 19 on Drug Dependence and Drug Abuse).

CHAPTER 13

Neurotoxics: Psychotropics and Designer Drugs

Classify the Psychotropic or Psychoactive agents with suitable examples?

Psychotropic agents are the substances or drugs that cause alterations in perception, mood, behavior, or consciousness. These are classified into four categories that are illustrated in Flowchart 1.

Flowchart 1: Classification of psychoactive agents

Classification of psychoactive agents

CNS depressants	CNS stimulants	Psychedelics/ Hallucinogens	Others (Medications)
– Alcohol (Date rape drugs)	– Cocaine	– Cannabis	– Antipsychotics
– GHB (Date rape drugs)	– Caffeine	– Datura	– Antidepressants
– Ketamine (Date rape drugs)	– Nicotine	– Psilocybin	– Mood stabilizers
– Inhalants	– Amphetamine	– Mescaline	– Disulfiram
– Opioids	– MDMA (Ecstasy) (Designer drug)	– LSD	– Naloxone, Naltrexone
– Sedatives/hypnotics		– Phencyclidine	– Methadone

Abbreviations: CNS, central nervous system; GHB, gamma-hydroxybutyric acid; LSD, Lysergic acid diethylamide; MDMA, 3,4-methhylenedioxymethamphetamine

Write a note on hallucinogens with a special reference to LSD and Phencyclidine?

Hallucinogens or psychedelics are agents that cause hallucinations at lower doses.

- *Action:* Alter the function of neurotransmitters especially serotonin.
- *Clinical manifestations:* Disordered thoughts, mood changes, dreamy state, disorientation, loss of contact with reality, hallucinations, etc.
- Hallucinogens cause marked *psychological dependence.*
- Some of the hallucinogens are lysergic acid diethylamide (LSD), phencyclidine, psilocybin (*hallucinogenic mushroom*), mescaline, etc.

Lysergic acid diethylamide (LSD)

Lysergic acid diethylamide was first synthesized from ergot alkaloids. Ergot contains ergotamine which is used in synthesis of LSD.

Note: Ergot fungus; e.g. Claviceps purpurea causes ergotism.

Route

Oral [rarely intramuscular (IM) or intravenous (IV)].

Action

Serotonin receptor agonist. LSD is one of the most potent hallucinogen, effective at very low doses.

Clinical manifestations

Dilated pupils, photophobia, tremors (within minutes), illusions, visual hallucinations (within 1–2 hours), tachycardia, hypertension, hyperthermia, feeling of detachment and derealization (life appears to be *like a movie*) and mood changes, etc.

Complications

- *Acute panic episodes* that may persist for 24 hours
- *Flash back phenomenon:* Recurrences of LSD experience occurs weeks to months after being in a drug free state
- Lysergic acid diethylamide is highly addictive and tolerance develops very rapidly
- *LSD dependence* is typically *psychological and not physical.* No withdrawal on stoppage.

Management

- Shift the patient to quite dark room
- Supportive treatment; reassurance and psychotherapy is the mainstay
- Benzodiazepines (for acute panic reactions).

Phencyclidine (angel dust)

Route

Sniffed, smoked, IV injections or orally.

Action

N-methyl-D-aspartate (NMDA) receptor antagonist.

Clinical manifestations

- Excitement, agitated behavior, flushing, sweating, dilated pupils, tremors, tachycardia, etc. *Presence of horizontal and vertical nystagmus is pathognomonic*
- Phencyclidine (PCP) is commonly associated with impaired judgment and reckless behavior
- *Phencyclidine overdose (at higher doses):* Marked hypertension, hyperthermia and seizures are reported.

Management

- Ventilatory support and benzodiazepines to control seizures
- Acidification of urine to enhance its excretion.

Write a note on designer drugs with a brief mention about MDMA?

Designer drugs

- Designer drugs are synthetic analogs of a controlled substances or prohibited drugs that have a slightly modified structure but pharmacological action similar to the prohibited drug
- Designer drugs are synthesized for recreational use circumventing the laws on illicit drugs

- Designer drugs typically have higher potency, longer duration of action and are difficult to detect
- Designer drugs are known to cause increased alertness, concentration, sexual stimulation, mood enhancement and euphoria, etc.
- The term designer drug was coined for analogs of fentanyl (synthetic opioid) also known as "China white", "drop dead", or "serial killer". The term, however, is more commonly related to analogs of amphetamines (methamphetamine), most popular being 3,4-methylenedioxymethamphetamine (MDMA) or ecstasy, 3,4-methylenedioxyamphetamine (MDA), etc.

Note: European Union has even included performance enhancing drugs such as synthetic steroids (commonly associated with doping in sports) as designer drugs.

- Newer designer drugs are called "legal highs" and include:
  - Substituted cathinones [*bath salts* that include mephedrone, methylenedioxypyrovalerone (MDPV) and methylone]
  - Synthetic cannabinoids (Brand names: K2, Spice, etc.)
  - Synthetic hallucinogens (derivative of phenethylamines; 25I-NBOMe, NBOMe, N-bomb).

Note: Cathinone is an alkaloid of plant Khat (Catha edulis) that has stimulant and euphoriant effects. The leaves of the plant are chewed as a social custom.

List of some of the common designer drugs thus include; MDMA (Ecstasy), Methylone, Mephedrone, and MDPV (each found in bath salts), K2 and Spice (synthetic cannabinoids), N-bomb, NBOMe (synthetic hallucinogens), and Krokodil (morphine derivative Desomorphine), etc.

Route of administration

Intranasal, oral, inhalation or by IV or IM injections.

Toxicity

Acute agitation is characteristic along with anxiety, tachycardia and psychosis.

Toxicity of designer drugs should be suspected in those presenting with acute neuropsychiatric complaints.

Management

Supportive (for both psychiatric and self-resolving nonpsychiatric symptoms) and symptomatic (benzodiazepines to treat anxiety, agitation and seizures).

Medicolegal aspects and circumstances of poisoning

- Accidental overdose and even mass fatalities are reported
- Detection is difficult (due to smaller doses, faster action and elimination)
- These are often associated with date rape or drug-facilitated sexual assaults (DFSAs).

MDMA/Ecstasy

3,4-methylenedioxymethamphetamine (MDMA or Ecstasy) is a designer drug that has gained notoriety for its abuse potential as a recreational drug (club drugs/rave drugs/party drugs) commonly taken by young students. MDMA has both central nervous system (CNS) stimulant and hallucinogenic effects, and is known to act as a sexual enhancer. Toxicity includes hyperthermia, cardiovascular instability, anxiety, acute panic attacks and seizures, etc.

Note: As much as 40% of the amphetamines are excreted unchanged in urine. The urine of amphetamine addicts is collected and sold on streets referred to as "**liquid gold**".

Write a short note on inhalant abuse/solvent abuse/glue sniffing?

Inhalant abuse/solvent abuse/glue sniffing/volatile substance misuse (VSM)

Volatile substances are abused by inhalation to produce feelings of euphoria. These include:

- *Gases including anesthetics:* Aerosols and sprays (deodorants and paint sprays), chloroform, diethyl ether, nitrous oxide, etc.
- *Industrial solvents:* Glues, paint thinners, varnishes, inks, shoe polish, aerosol products, kerosene, gasoline, etc.
- *Organic nitrites:* Amyl nitrite, isobutyl nitrite, etc. known as "poppers".

Initially glue (a toluene based adhesive) was abused in sniffing hence, the name glue sniffing.

Methods of inhalation

- *Bagging:* A bag containing volatile solvents is put around mouth and nostrils and inhaled
- *Dusting:* Spraying the volatile substance directly in the mouth or nostrils
- *Glading:* Spraying the room with the volatile substance followed by deep inspiration
- *Huffing:* Cloth pad is moistened with the substance and kept over mouth (oral inhalation)
- *Sniffing or snorting:* Inhalation of fumes directly from the container (nasal inhalation).

Intoxicating symptoms

Dreamy state, hallucinations, euphoria, behavioral changes, etc.

Cause of death

Cardiac arrhythmias, hypoxia or anoxia or plastic bag asphyxia.

CHAPTER 14

Neurotoxics: Spinal Poisons

Classify spinal poisons?

Spinal poisons act mainly on the spinal cord. Based on its manifestations these are classified as:

Stimulant spinal poisons	*Depressant spinal poisons*
Causes spasm and convulsions	Causes paralysis and loss of sensation
For example *Strychnos nux-vomica* (*Kuchila*)	For example *Gelsemium sempervirens*
	Physostigmatis semina (*Calabar beans*)

Enumerate the active principles of Strychnos nux-vomica (Kuchila, dog buttons). Write a detailed note on Strychnine poisoning including its mechanism of action, clinical manifestations, management, postmortem findings and medicolegal significance?

Strychnos nux-vomica

Active principles include:

- Strychnine (principle alkaloid), brucine (alkaloid), loganin (glucoside).
- Strychnine is obtained from the seeds of *Strychnos nux-vomica* and is 10–20 times more potent than brucine that is contained in the bark, leaves, etc.
- Strychnine is available as a white crystalline odorless powder that is bitter in taste.

Mechanism of action

Site of action

Anterior horn cells of the spinal cord. It primarily affects the motor nerves in the spinal cord which control muscle contraction.

Strychnine acts as an antagonist of inhibitory neurotransmitter glycine. It blocks the receptors preventing the postsynaptic uptake of glycine by brain stem and spinal cord. The widespread inhibition results in increased reflex excitability.

Fatal dose

1–3 crushed seeds (intact seeds are harmless) or 20–50 mg of strychnine.

Fatal period

1–2 hours.

Clinical Manifestations

Clinical manifestations of strychnine poisoning can be remembered by the **mnemonic:** ***(A–H O–T)*:**

A:	Anxiety, Apprehension
B:	Bitter taste, Bow-shaped body
C:	Choking sensation, Convulsions, Cyanosis, Consciousness retained
D:	Dysphagia, Dilated pupils, Death is painful due to respiratory arrest
E:	Epigastric pain, *Emprosthotonus* i.e. forward arching of the body may occur rarely (Fig. 1)
F:	Froth, Fear of impending death
G:	Glycine antagonist
H:	Hyperthermia, *Hippus* (spasmodic pupil is classically associated with aconite)
O:	*Opisthotonus,* i.e. backward arching of the body; body in supine position rests on head and heels (Fig. 1)
P:	Painful muscle spasm, *Pleurothotonus,* i.e. sideways arching of the body may occur rarely (Fig. 1)
Q:	Kidney and liver injury
R:	*Risus sardonicus* (grinning expression or involuntary smile as the angles of mouth are drawn backwards due to sustained spasm of facial muscles), Restlessness
S:	*Satan's face or sardonic grin* (devilish grin), Spasm of muscles
T:	*Trismus* or lock jaw, Twitching and tremor of muscles, *Tetanus like symptoms*

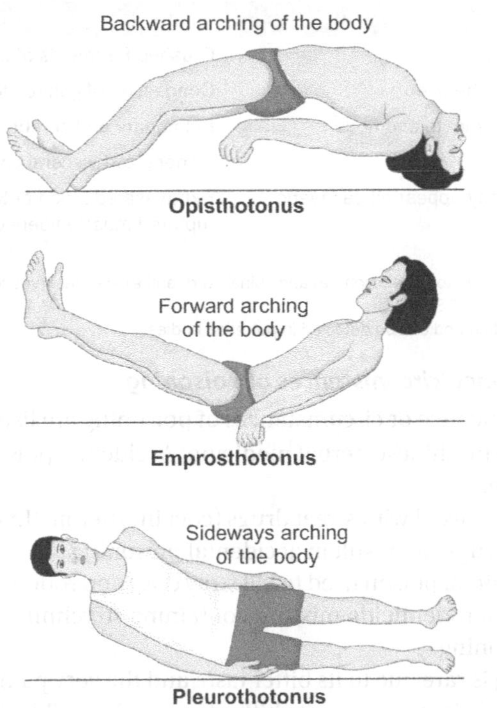

Fig. 1: Arching of the body in strychnine poisoning

Management

- Good supportive care (maintain airway, breathing and circulation).
- Prevention and treatment of convulsions is the mainstay of treatment:
  - Keep the patient in quiet and dark room.
  - Intravenous (IV) administration of short-acting barbiturates or diazepam with short-acting muscle relaxants.
- Decontamination:
  - Gastric lavage with potassium permanganate ($KMnO_4$) should be attempted only after convulsions are controlled.
- Symptomatic treatment
- Morphine is contraindicated (may precipitate convulsions, and worsen respiratory insufficiency).

Cause of death

Respiratory failure due to prolonged spasm of respiratory muscles or occasionally from exhaustion.

Postmortem appearances

The specific postmortem observations in fatal strychnine poisoning are illustrated in Table 1.

Table 1: Postmortem appearances in fatal strychnine poisoning

External examination	*Internal examination*
Rigor mortis appears early	Crushed fragments of seed in the stomach
Postmortem caloricity may be seen	Congestion of gastrointestinal mucosa
Froth (blood stained) from mouth and nose	Pulmonary and cerebral edema
Cyanosis of extremities	Generalized visceral congestion
Extreme muscle rigidity may appear as cadaveric spasm	Extravasated blood between muscle fibers (due to ruptured muscle fibers during spasm)

Note

- Apart from routine viscera, brain (one hemisphere) and spinal cord (entire) are preserved for chemical analysis at the Regional Forensic Science Laboratory (RFSL).
- Strychnine resists putrefaction and can be detected in putrefied bodies.

Medicolegal significance/circumstances of poisoning

The medicolegal significance or circumstances of poisoning are listed as follows:

- Strychnine is used in Chinese herbal medicine. Accidental poisoning may occur due to its therapeutic misuse.
- Strychnine is rarely mixed with street drugs (cocaine/heroin/LSD). Smoking or snorting of such adulterated drugs can result in accidental poisoning.
- Strychnine is an animal poison used to kill stray dogs and rodents (rodenticide). Accidental or suicidal intake of rodenticide mixture containing strychnine remains a common cause of strychnine poisoning.
- Suicidal poisoning is rare due to its bitter taste and the very painful death it causes.
- Homicidal poisoning is rare due to its bitter taste and possible detection even in putrefied bodies.
- Tolerance develops on repetitive intake of small doses.

Give the differential diagnosis for strychnine poisoning and mention the differentiating features of tetanus and strychnine poisoning?

Differential diagnosis

Clinical manifestations of Strychnine poisoning are similar to:

- Epileptic fits (differentiating features include; history of epilepsy, loss of consciousness is present, and recovery is spontaneous).
- Tetanus (differentiating features of tetanus and strychnine poisoning are shown in Table 2).

Table 2: Differentiating features of tetanus and strychnine poisoning

Features	*Strychnine poisoning*	*Tetanus*
History	Poisoning	Injury
Mechanism of action	Blocks the uptake of glycine	Blocks the release of glycine
Onset of symptoms	Sudden (in 15 min–1 hour)	Gradual
Convulsions	Generalized (all muscles affected at the same time)	Non-generalized (neck muscles are affected first followed by lock jaw)
Trismus or lock jaw	May be a late feature	Appears early (involves lower jaw)
State of muscles	Relaxed between convulsions	In spasm throughout
Course of disease	Steady (improves or worsens)	Not steady
Death	Within a few hours	Delayed for days
Chemical analysis	Positive for strychnine	Negative
Microbiology	Negative	Positive for *Clostridium tetani*

CHAPTER 15

Cardiac Poisons

Enumerate some cardiotoxic plants and their active principles.

Some of the cardiotoxic plants and their active principles are listed in Table 1.

Table 1: Cardiotoxic plants and their active principles

Plant	Common names	Active principles
*Nicotiana tabacum**	Tobacco, tambaku	Nicotine, anabasine, nicotianine, lobeline
Nerium oleander *Nerium odorum*	Common or Pink oleander, kaner, dog bane	Nerine, nerioside, folinerin, rosagenin, oleandrin
Cerbera thevetia *Thevetia peruviana*	Pila kaner, lucky nut, yellow oleander	Cerberin, thevetin, thevetoxin, nerifolin
Cerbera odollam	Pilikirbir, suicide tree	Cerberin, odollin, odolotoxin, thevetin
Aconitum ferox *Aconitum napellus*	Aconite, mitha zaher, bish, bikh, monk's hood	Aconitine, mesaconitine, hypaconitine, bikhaconitine, indaconitine, picraconitine
Digitalis purpurea	Common foxglove	Digitoxin, digitalin, digoxin
Cinchona officinalis	Quinine, fever tree	Quinine, Quinidine, Cinchonine

***Note:** Fatal dose of nicotine is 50–100 mg; for crude tobacco the fatal dose is 15–30 grams.

See pictures of *Nerium*, *Cerbera thevetia*, *Cerbera odollam*, and aconite root in Chapter 26 on Appliances and Spotters in Practical Examinations.

Write a note on aconitine (aconite) poisoning?

Aconitine (aconite) poisoning

Mechanism of action

Aconitine and other alkaloids of aconite bind to the voltage-sensitive sodium channels of the myocardium, nerves and muscles causing a persistent activation of the sodium channels. Aconite thus, has *cardiotoxic and neurotoxic* propensity. Vagal activity of aconitine and related alkaloids is responsible for its arrhythmogenic properties.

Clinical manifestations

Clinical manifestations of aconitine poisoning are illustrated in Table 2.

Characteristic symptoms of aconitine poisoning

The characteristic symptoms of aconitine poisoning are given as follows:

- Tingling followed by numbness and burning sensation of the face that spreads all over the body gradually.

Table 2: Clinical manifestations of aconitine poisoning

Neurological features (within 10–20 minutes)	*Gastrointestinal features (within 2–6 hours)*	*Cardiovascular features (within 8–12 hours)*
Tingling, numbness and burning sensation of mouth, lips, tongue and throat. Weakness and pain in limb muscles (convulsions may be a late feature)	Nausea, vomiting, and pain abdomen. Colicky diarrhea follows	Hypotension, bradycardia and cardiac rhythm disturbances (sinus tachycardia, ventricular tachycardia and ventricular fibrillation, etc.)

- No loss of consciousness (since aconitine does not affect the higher centers of brain).
- *Hippus or spasmodic pupil* (referred to as alternate constriction and dilatation of pupils). See chapter 3 '*General Principles of Toxicology*' for detailed description of hippus.
- ***Xanthopsia*** *or yellow vision:* Patient at times complains of seeing yellow halos around objects.

Fatal dose
3–6 mg of aconitine.

Fatal period
12–24 hours.

Causes of death
Ventricular arrhythmias and asystole, respiratory failure.

Management
- Decontamination [gastric lavage with potassium permanganate ($KMnO_4$)].
- Symptomatic and supportive treatment as there is no specific antidote.
- Bradycardia is treated with atropine and intravenous (IV) fluids are administered for treating hypotension.

Medicolegal significance and circumstances of poisoning
The circumstances of aconitine poisoning are described as follows:
- *Accidental poisoning:* It may occur when the root of aconite that is the most toxic part of the plant is *mistaken for horse radish* (an ingredient used in preparation of sauce) due to their close resemblance.
- *Suicidal poisoning:* It is rarely reported.
- Aconite is often considered as an *ideal homicidal poison* due to its following properties:
  - Its taste can be easily masked by mixing it with alcohol, sweets or betel leaves
  - Quick acting and fatal in small doses (high toxicity)
  - Death is quick and appears as sudden cardiac death (arrhythmias)
  - Difficulty in detection: Aconite alkaloids are destroyed quickly in human body and by putrefaction.
- Used in the past as abortifacient, arrow and cattle or animal poison.
- Aconite as *warfare agent*:
  - Used as an *arrow poison* during wars in ancient times.
  - Aconitine-treated bullets were tested by the Nazis during the World War II.

Note: In a suspected or alleged case of aconite poisoning, heart and brain should be preserved along with the routine viscera, for chemical analysis at the Regional Forensic Science Laboratory (RFSL). Viscera is to be preserved in rectified spirit and not in saturated solution of common salt.

CHAPTER 16

Asphyxiants: Respiratory Poisons

Classification of asphyxiants

Classification of asphyxiants

Simple asphyxiants	Chemical asphyxiants	Respiratory irritants	Others
Act mechanically – N_2 – CH_4 – Inert gases	Prevent O_2 utilization – CO – CO_2 – HCN – H_2S	Irritation of air passages – Tear gas – Phosgene – NH_3, Cl_2, NO_2, SO_2, etc.	Systemic poisons Anesthetic agents

Write a note on carbon monoxide (CO) poisoning?

Carbon monoxide is a colorless, odorless, tasteless and non-irritant gas that is rapidly absorbed by the lungs.

Mechanism of action

- The affinity of CO to hemoglobin (Hb) is 200–250 times greater than oxygen. Hence, it readily binds to Hb and forms carboxyhemoglobin (COHb) resulting in *anemic anoxia/hypoxia.*
- Likewise, CO also binds to myoglobin (60 times greater affinity than O_2). With increasing levels of COHb, there is a leftward shift of the oxyhemoglobin dissociation curve. CO also affects the intracellular respiration by blocking cytochrome oxidase and cytochrome P450, etc.

Clinical manifestations

Vary with the COHb concentrations, and are described in Table 1.

Table 1: Clinical manifestations of carbon monoxide poisoning corresponding to varying carboxyhemoglobin (COHb) levels

COHb%	*Clinical manifestations*
0–10	Asymptomatic
10–20	Mild headache, breathlessness on exertion
20–30	Throbbing headache, irritability, fatigue, emotional instability

Contd...

Contd...

COHb%	Clinical manifestations
30–40	Severe headache, nausea, vomiting, dizziness, dimness of vision, tinnitus, confusion, and cherry red discoloration of skin
40–50	Increasing confusion, ataxia, rapid respiration, hallucinations, muscle incoordination Symptoms resemble alcohol intoxication
50–60	Pink or red discoloration of skin, rapid respiration, tachycardia, convulsions, and coma
>60	Skin blisters (cutaneous bullae), deep coma, arrhythmias, and death

Note: The COHb levels may not always correlate with clinical findings and symptoms. Patients with pre-existing cardiac or lung disease, fetus, infants, or elderly are affected relatively more due to their limited capacity to tolerate cardiovascular compromise.

Delayed neurological and neuropsychiatric effects such as impaired memory, mood and personality changes may be observed after days of CO exposure.

Fatal dose
COHb > 60%

Fatal period
Within few hours

Cause of death
Respiratory arrest

Diagnosis

- Raised levels of carboxyhemogloin (COHb) in blood
- Quantitative analysis is recommended as the COHb levels are raised in smokers (Nonsmokers have COHb levels of 1%, whereas smokers have COHb levels ranging between 4% and 10%).

Note: In cases of death due to burns, raised COHb levels at autopsy are indicative of antemortem burns.

Treatment

- Removal from the source. Assisted ventilation.
- Administration of 100% oxygen
- Hyperbaric oxygen when COHb levels are more than 25%.

Postmortem appearances

Observations at postmortem examination are described in Table 2.

Table 2: Postmortem appearances in carbon monoxide poisoning

External examination	Internal examination
Cherry red appearance of postmortem staining	Cherry red appearance of internal organs
Skin blisters (cutaneous bullae)	Pulmonary and cerebral edema
Froth at the mouth and nostrils	Softening of basal ganglia in delayed deaths

*Apart from routine viscera, lungs are preserved for chemical analysis at the Regional Forensic Science Laboratory (RFSL)

Medicolegal significance and circumstances of carbon monoxide poisoning

- *Accidental poisonings*
  - Carbon monoxide in large amounts causes rapid death as the victim is unable to notice this deadly colorless, odorless, tasteless and nonirritant gas
  - Accidental exposures may occur in house fires, and fires/smoke in confined spaces.
  - Accidental exposures are due to defective heating appliances (gas geysers, fire places, chimneys, etc.) especially in poorly ventilated and confined spaces.
  - Accidental poisoning has been reported in cars with the engine running for long hours due to obstructed tail pipe and/or defective exhaust system that results in CO accumulation.
  - Carbon monoxide poisoning has also been reported in hookah smoking.
- *Suicidal poisonings*
  - Carbon monoxide is an effective method of suicide as it causes painless and rapid death.
  - Charcoal burning in confined spaces is used as an easy and painless method of suicide in Japan.
  - Carbon monoxide has been found to be the cause for *car-running-in-garage suicides* in the past. These suicides were practiced by running the car engine in a garage or any similar nonventilated space for long hours, or by keeping the engine running and putting an exhaust hosepipe into the car through the window. Accumulation of deadly exhaust fumes containing CO causes rapid death.
- *Carbon monoxide poisoning is a difficult diagnosis.* Mild CO poisoning resembles flu-like syndromes and can be misdiagnosed as migraine, chronic fatigue, depression, etc. While symptoms of moderate to severe CO poisoning are similar to alcohol intoxication, CVA, and epilepsy, etc.
- *Phosgene,* a war gas (respiratory irritant) is carbonyl chloride (a combination of CO and Cl_2).

Write a brief note on "Ghost wells/Haunted wells"?

Carbon dioxide (CO_2) is formed due to decay of organic matter in the bottom of unused tanks or wells, and stays there since it is heavier than the air. Unsuspecting workers/cleaners are accidentally exposed to the toxic CO_2 as they reach the bottom of an unused well or tank. Death is very quick and occurs due to lack of oxygen (asphyxia). At times such wells are referred as "Ghost wells". CO_2 results in hypoxic hypoxia in contrast to CO that causes anemic hypoxia (Table 3).

Table 3: Clinical manifestations of carbon dioxide poisoning

Blood CO_2 concentrations	*Clinical manifestations*
2–5%	Throbbing headache
>5%	Toxic effects; increased respiratory rate, dizziness, visual and hearing impairment, unconsciousness
>10%	Convulsions, coma and death

Write a note on hydrocyanic acid (prussic acid)/hydrogen cyanide (HCN) poisoning?

Hydrocyanic acid is a liquid, while hydrogen cyanide is a colorless gas, also referred as hydrocyanic gas.

Cyanide salts (sodium cyanide, potassium cyanide, etc.) occur in solid state as white powders.

Cyanides generally produce a characteristic bitter almond odor. The bitter almond odor can be perceived by about 60–70% of the human population, and the ability to do so is a sex-linked recessive trait.

Mechanism of action

- Cyanide is rapidly absorbed through all routes after exposure. When ingested, cyanide salts are converted to lethal hydrogen cyanide by the action of hydrochloric acid released in stomach.
  Achlorhydrics, thus, are relatively protected from the toxic effects of cyanide salts.
  NaCN/KCN + HCl → HCN + NaCl/KCl
- Likewise, water in the gastric juice can hydrolyze cyanide salts to lethal hydrogen cyanide.
  NaCN/KCN + H2O → HCN + NaOH/KOH
- Hydrogen cyanide is a metabolic poison. Cyanide ions combine with, and inhibits enzyme systems of cellular respiration such as cytochrome oxidase, carbonic anhydrase, etc. Large doses of cyanide causes *histotoxic anoxia* (i.e. prevents cells from using oxygen). Cyanide poisoning results in increased levels of oxyhemoglobin in venous blood and also the levels of lactic acid.
- The major part of the HCN is metabolized by the enzyme Rhodanase and excreted in urine as nontoxic thiocyanates. Remaining part is excreted unchanged in breath (bitter almond odor).
  $\text{HCN} \xrightarrow{\text{Rhodanase/Thiosulfate}}$ Thiocyanate (nontoxic) excreted by kidneys

Clinical manifestations

Depends on the route of administration (very rapid if inhaled than on ingestion), dose and duration of exposure.

- *Ingestion*: Burning pain in the mouth, throat and stomach, nausea, and bitter almond odor in breath.
- *Dermal contact*: Irritant dermatitis/"cyanide rash" (itching, vesication and skin disruption).
- *General symptoms*: Headache, vertigo, weakness, anxiety, confusion, difficulty in breathing, dilated pupils, tachycardia, hypotension, convulsions and loss of consciousness.

Clinical manifestations vary with the blood cyanide concentrations (mg/dL) and are described in Table 4.

Table 4: Clinical manifestations of cyanide poisoning

Blood cyanide level (mg/dL)	*Clinical manifestations*
0.20–0.30	Respiratory depression, Coma
>0.30	Death

Fatal dose

Pure HCN = 50–100 mg; NaCN/KCN = 200–300 mg

Fatal period

Pure HCN = 2–10 minutes; NaCN/KCN = 30 minutes

Cause of death

Respiratory arrest, cardiac arrhythmias

Diagnosis

Based on cyanide levels in whole blood by gas chromatography/spectrophotometry.

Lee Jones test is a rapid bedside test

5 mL of gastric aspirate + few Fe_2SO_4 crystals + 5 drops of NaOH solution ⇒ Boil, then cool and add few drops of 10% HCl ⇒ Greenish blue precipitate shows presence of cyanide.

Note: Purplish precipitate in Lee Jones test indicates presence of salicylates.

Treatment

- Shift the victim to fresh air. Remove the contaminated clothing.
- *Dermal/Ocular exposure*: Wash the skin and eyes with large amounts of water.
- In cases of ingestion, gastric lavage with sodium thiosulfate solution is useful.
- Give 100% oxygen therapy (*reverses binding of cyanide to cytochrome oxidase sites*).
- *Antidotal therapy (Eli-Lilly cyanide antidote kit/three-step cyanide antidote kit)*: It is meant to *interfere with the binding of cyanide to cytochrome oxidase system and facilitate its excretion (Table 5 and Fig. 1).*

Table 5: Three-step cyanide antidote kit

First step	*Second step*	*Third step*
Amyl nitrite inhalation (0.3 ml ampoule is broken and inhaled for 30 seconds)	3% *sodium nitrite* solution (10 ml slow IV injection for 5 minutes)	25% *sodium thiosulfate* solution (50 ml IV infusion over 10–20 minutes)
Nitrites induce methemoglobin formation that has higher affinity for CN than cytochrome oxidase; the CN ions get dissociated from cyanide cytochrome oxidase complex and form a relatively nontoxic cyanmethemoglobin.		*Cyanide is excreted as nontoxic thiocyanate due to action of thiosulfate in the presence of enzyme rhodanase.*

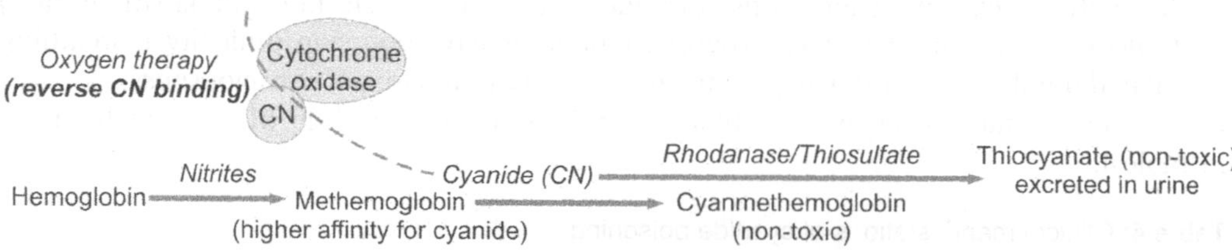

Fig. 1: Antidotal therapy in cyanide poisoning

Alternate therapy

- *4-dimethylaminophenol (DMAP)*: Methemoglobin-inducing agent (as an alternate to nitrites).
- *Dicobalt edetate*: As an alternate to other methemoglobin-inducing agents.
- *Hydroxocobalamin (IV infusion)*: With cyanide nontoxic cyanocobalamin is formed (excreted).
- Symptomatic treatment (vasopressors for hypotension and sodium bicarbonate to treat acidosis).

Note: Methylene blue is used to treat methemoglobinemia (can cause blue urine discoloration). Reddish discoloration of urine is reported in hydroxocobalamin treatment of CN poisoning.

Postmortem appearances

Postmortem findings in fatal cyanide poisoning are shown in Table 6.

Table 6: Postmortem observations in cyanide poisoning

External examination	*Internal examination*
Brick red appearance of postmortem staining	Pinkish red appearance of internal organs
Skin blisters, dilated pupils	Bitter almond odor in gastric contents
Fine froth at the mouth and nostrils.	Pulmonary and cerebral edema

*Apart from routine viscera, lungs and spleen are preserved for chemical analysis at the Regional Forensic Science Laboratory (RFSL)

Medicolegal significance/Circumstances of cyanide poisoning:

- *Unintentional exposure*
  - People may be exposed to low levels of cyanides routinely from cigarette smoke, vehicle exhaust, combustion products, or consumption of fruits/vegetables containing cyanide.
  - A glycoside amygdalin is present in bitter almonds, peach, apricot, cherry and plum, etc. which contains cyanide (cyanogenic glycoside). Cyanide is released from amygdalin due to the action of enzyme emulsion causing its poisoning.
  - Accidental exposure can occur to the handlers/technicians in their dealing with:
    - ◊ 4% hydrocyanic acid solution known as "Scheele's acid" that is used in veterinary practice.
    - ◊ Cyanide salts that are used as common laboratory reagents
    - ◊ Cyanide and cyanide-containing compounds that are used for fumigation, plastic manufacturing, electroplating, and photodeveloping, and by goldsmiths in India for gold plating.
  - Smoke inhalation during house or industrial fires can be a major source of cyanide poisoning.
  - Cyanide is a potential health hazard for forensic pathologists and mortuary staff. During autopsies on victims who have consumed large amounts of cyanide salts, evolving hydrogen cyanide gas in the stomach can cause poisoning to the mortuary staffers during examination of gastric contents.
- *Intentional exposure*: Cyanide is a rapidly acting and highly lethal poison. Its intentional use is reported as a warfare agent/as an agent for judicial execution/or to commit suicide/ homicide.

  Chemical warfare: Cyanides have the potential to be used as agents of terrorism. Historically, World War I saw their use as chemical weapons for the first time.
  - *Gas chambers*: Hydrogen cyanide gas is used to execute death sentence.
  - *Cyanide pills and vials* have been used to commit suicide by terrorists/criminals to escape interrogation. It was a common method employed by the LTTE members who used to wear cyanide vials around their necks and consume it on being caught by the forces.
  - *Mass suicides and genocide*: Cyanide was used by the Nazis for the aforementioned purposes.
  - *"Goldsmith suicides"*: In India, a number of goldsmiths have reportedly committed suicide by consuming cyanide that is cheap and easily available to them for its use in gold plating.

  - *Homicide*: Cases of homicide by administering cyanide are reported from India and abroad. Kempamma @ Mallika, a woman serial killer used cyanide to murder 11 women in Karnataka, India.
- *Postmortem production of cyanide*: Cyanide may be produced postmortem due to decomposition. Hence, careful interpretation of analytical observations is mandatory.

Write a brief note on hydrogen sulfide (H_2S) poisoning?

Hydrogen sulfide is an irritant and a chemical asphyxiant. It acts by cytochrome oxidase inhibition.

Clinical manifestations

Route of poisoning is inhalational. Signs of ocular and respiratory irritation, headache, vertigo, respiratory depression, arrhythmias, and coma are seen.

Treatment

- Shift the victim to fresh air
- 100% oxygen therapy is the mainstay of treatment
- Supportive and symptomatic care.
- **Antidotes:** *Amyl nitrite and sodium nitrite* (similar to treatment for cyanide poisoning except that thiosulfate is not used). *Nitrites induce methemoglobin formation (as described in cyanide poisoning). H_2S readily combines with methemoglobin to form sulfmethemoglobin.*

Cause of death

Respiratory arrest, cardiac arrhythmias

Postmortem observations

- Characteristic smell of "rotten eggs" around the mouth and nostrils
- Presence of fine froth in the airways, mouth and nostrils
- Partial greenish discoloration of the skin, airways, and viscera especially the lungs and the brain surface has been reported.
- Marked pulmonary and cerebral edema is evident in almost all cases.
- Raised thiosulfate levels in the blood, brain and lungs are confirmatory.

Medicolegal significance

Hydrogen sulfide is a rapidly acting and highly lethal poison. Poisoning is mostly accidental and reported among sewage/septic tank cleaners (sewer gas). At high concentrations, the ability to identify H_2S by its characteristic "rotten egg" odor vanishes due to "olfactory fatigue" and the victim collapses/loses consciousness rapidly.

Suicidal cases too have been reported.

Note: ***Sewer gas*** is a mixture of gases including H_2S, CH_4, NH_3, CO, SO_2, etc.

CHAPTER 17

Warfare Agents

What are warfare agents? Classify and briefly describe its types.

Warfare agents are used for destruction or damage of human lives mostly in times of war.

Warfare agents are classified as:

- *Biological warfare agents*: Biological warfare agents include microorganisms or their product of metabolism/toxins with an ability to infect and grow in the target host producing a clinical disease that kills or incapacitates. Various bacteria, viruses and fungi can be used as infectious agents/toxins in biological warfare, e.g. anthrax spores and botulinum toxins.
- *Chemical warfare agents*: Chemical warfare agents are any substance solid, liquid or gas intended to cause harm/destruction of human population in the times of war, e.g. war gases. These are usually referred to as "gas" irrespective of their state.

Agents such as tear gas and low-risk sternutators are also used to disperse disruptive mob during riots and referred to as riot control agents (RCAs). Commonly employed RCAs nowadays are Chloroacetophenone (CN) gas, ortho-chlorobenzylidene-malononitrile (CS) gas*, diphenylamine chlorarsine (DM), pepper sprays, tasers, rubber bullets, etc.

Write a note on bioterrorism and biological warfare agents?

Bioterrorism is the intentional release of biological warfare agents causing large scale human morbidity and mortality. Biological warfare agents are described in Table 1.

Table 1: Categorization of biological warfare agents and their properties

Category	Properties	Agents (Diseases)
Category A	• Maximum adverse public health impact • Mass casualties • High potential of large scale dissemination and panic among public	• *Clostridium botulinum* toxin (Botulism) • *Bacillus anthracis* (Anthrax) • *Yersinia pestis* (Plague) • *Variola major* (Smallpox) • *Francisella tularensis* (Tularemia) • Ebola virus, Lassa virus, etc. (Viral hemorrhagic fevers)

Contd...

Contd...

Category	*Properties*	*Agents (Diseases)*
Category B	• Lower public health impact • Lesser casualties • Lesser potential of large scale dissemination and panic among public • Agents causing food and water safety threats	• *Coxiella burnetii* (Q fever) • *Chlamydia psittaci* (Psittacosis) • *Brucella species* (Brucellosis) • *Rickettsia* species (Typhus fever) • Phytotoxins; Ricin and Abrin (Toxic syndromes) • Staphylococcal enterotoxin B (Toxic syndromes) • Alphaviruses (Viral encephalitis) • Food safety threats; *Salmonella, Escherichia coli* • Water safety threats; *Vibrio cholera*
Category C	• Potential of future threats from emerging agents • Capable of causing high morbidity and mortality	• *SARS (severe acute respiratory syndrome) coronavirus* • Influenza A virus (H1N1) • Nipah virus (Encephalitis) • *Hantavirus* (Hantavirus pulmonary syndrome)

Write a note on war gases?

Classification and characteristic symptoms of war gases have been explained in Table 2.

Table 2: Classification and characteristic symptoms of war gases

Class	*Agents*	*Characteristic symptoms*
Lachrymators (Tear gas*)	• Chloroacetophenone (CN gas) • Bromobenzyl cyanide (BBC) • Ethyliodoacetate (KSK)	• Extreme ocular irritation, flow of tears, spasm of eyelids and temporary blindness. • Skin blisters and irritation of air passages
Vesicants (Blistering gas)	• Mustard gas • Lewisite • Sulfur	• Irritation of skin, eyes, nose, and air passages. Nausea, vomiting, and abdominal pain. • Itching, vesication and ulceration of skin
Asphyxiants (Lung irritants) (Chocking gas)	• Chlorine • Phosgene, diphosgene • Chloropicrin	• Cough, dyspnea, tightness of chest, difficulty in breathing and cyanosis • Death due to acute pulmonary edema.
Sternutators (Nasal irritants) (Sickening gas)	• Diphenyl chlorarsine (DA) • Diphenyl cyanarsine (DC) • Diphenylamine chlorarsine (DM)	• These compounds of arsenic cause nasal/sinus irritation, sneezing, nausea, vomiting and tightness of chest.
Nerve gases	Tabun, Soman, Sarin	Act by inactivation of cholinesterase enzyme similar to organophosphates.
Paralysants	Carbon monoxide, hydrogen sulfide, and hydrocyanic acid	Described in detail in chapter 16 on asphyxiants

*Tear gas used globally nowadays is ortho-chlorobenzylidene-malononitrile (CS gas).

Management

- Remove the patient to fresh air and wash the affected parts thoroughly.
- Eyes should be washed with warm normal saline/boric acid/sodium bicarbonate solution.
- Supportive and antibiotic therapy.

CHAPTER 18
Agrochemicals

Classify agrochemicals/pesticides and name some compounds belonging to each group?

Classification of agrochemicals and pesticides has been described in Flowchart 1.

Flowchart 1: Classification of agrochemicals and pesticides

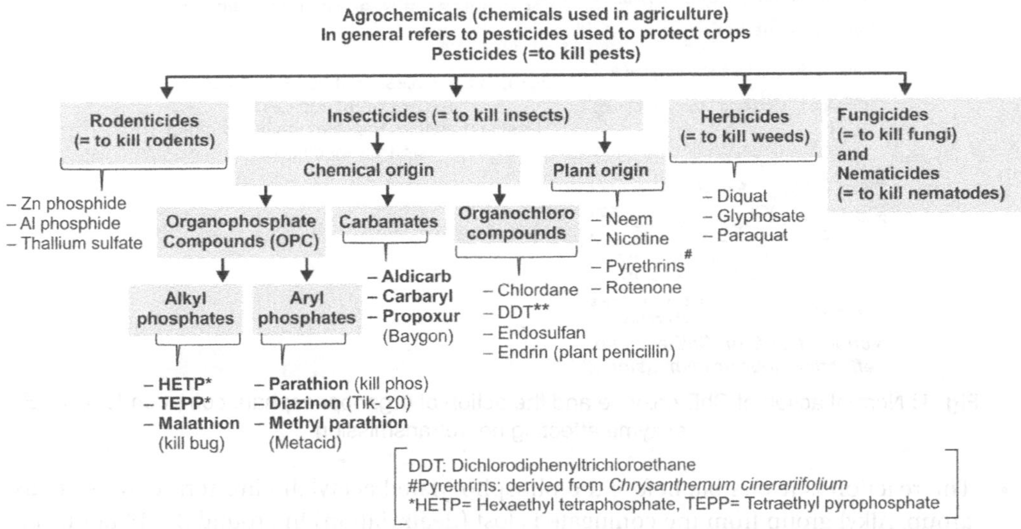

Describe in detail about organophosphate compound toxicity including its mechanism of action, clinical manifestations, management, postmortem findings and medicolegal significance?

Mechanism of action

Normal release and deactivation of acetylcholine (ACh): ACh is released in the synaptic cleft, and acts on the ACh receptors for transmission of impulse. cholinesterase (ChE) enzyme is responsible for the quick breakdown of ACh by hydrolysis into choline which is transported back to axon terminal (Fig. 1).

Action of organophosphate compounds (OPCs)

OPCs act by inhibition of cholinesterase (ChE) enzyme

(OPCs = cholinesterase inhibitors or anticholinesterases)

- The phosphate group of organophosphates combines with ChE enzyme; acetylcholinesterase (AChE or true cholinesterase) as well as butyrylcholinesterase (BuChE or pseudocholinesterase) resulting in *phosphorylation of the enzyme.* This phosphate-enzyme conjugate (phosphorylated acetylcholinesterase) is very stable, and thus, the degradation of ACh does not take place, which in turn leads to excess accumulation of ACh causing overstimulation of ACh receptors (Fig. 1).

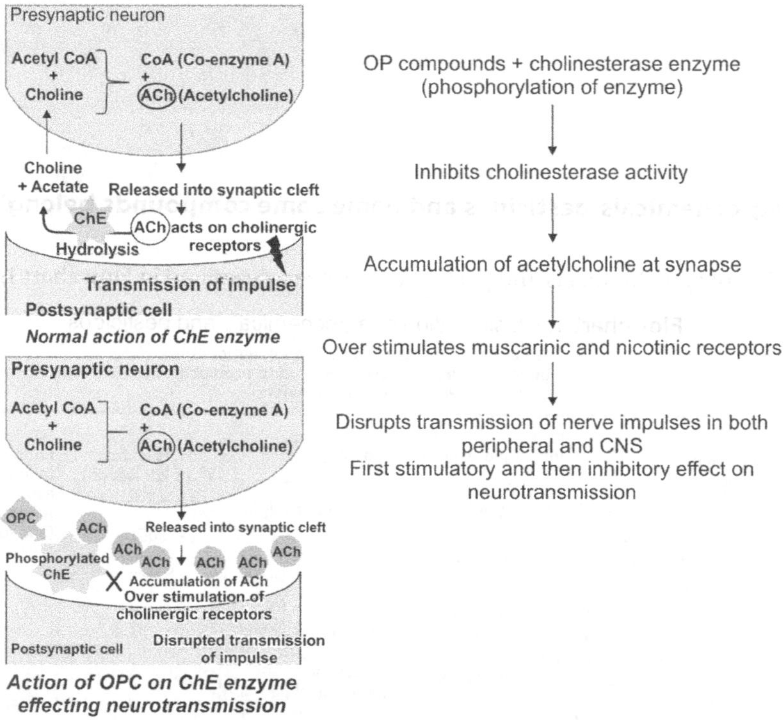

Fig. 1: Normal action of ChE enzyme and the action of organophosphate compounds on ChE enzyme affecting neurotransmission

- The reaction is reversible before the phosphorylated acetylcholinesterase loses an alkyl group. Alkyl group from the conjugate is lost (dealkylation) in around 24–48 hours, after which the enzyme becomes permanently inactivated. This process is known as *"Aging".*

Note: Aging of phosphorylated enzymes cannot be reversed by oximes. *Aging is not associated with carbamate poisoning.*

Organophosphate compounds are readily absorbed from intact skin, mucous membranes, conjunctiva, gastrointestinal and respiratory tracts, and are rapidly distributed to all body tissues. Most of the OPCs are highly lipid soluble and easily cross the blood-brain barrier.

Clinical manifestations

Clinical manifestations are described as muscarinic, nicotinic and central nervous system (CNS) effects (Flowchart 2).

- *Muscarinic effects* **[Mnemonic: *DUMBBELS*]:**
  - *Cardiovascular*: Bradycardia, hypotension
  - *Respiratory*: Rhinorrhea, bronchorrhea, bronchospasm, and cough
  - *Gastrointestinal*: Nausea/vomiting, abdominal cramps, diarrhea, and fecal incontinence
  - *Genitourinary*: Urinary incontinence
  - *Ocular*: Miosis (constricted pupils), blurred vision, and increased lacrimation
  - *Glands*: Excessive secretions, increased salivation, lacrimation, sweating, etc.

Note: Chromodacryorrhea (Red tears/Bloody tears/Colored tears) is often reported as a distinct feature of OP poisoning. Chromodacryorrhea, in fact, is predominantly reported in rats, and occurs due to muscarinic receptor stimulation causing release of porphyrin pigment by harderian glands located in the orbits of the animals. It is not a feature of human toxicity.

- *Nicotinic effects* **[Mnemonic: *MATCH*]:**
  - *Sympathetic ganglia*: Tachycardia and hypertension
  - *Musculoskeletal*: Fasciculation, weakness, cramps, and paralysis
- *CNS effects*:
  - *Early* **[Mnemonic: *RASH CAT*]:** Anxiety, restlessness, headache, confusion, ataxia, slurred speech, and tremors.
  - *Late* **[Mnemonic: *ARC CC*]:** Respiratory and circulatory depression, areflexia (absent reflexes), convulsions, and coma.

Neurological manifestations of organophosphate poisoning are summarized in Table 1.

Cause of death: Respiratory failure.

Flowchart 2: Clinical manifestations of organophosphate poisoning

Clinical manifestations of organophosphate poisoning

Muscarinic symptoms [DUMBBELS]	Nicotinic effects [MATCH]	CNS effects [Early effects: RASH CAT]
D: Diarrhea	M: Muscle fasciculation and spasm	R: Restlessness
U: Urinary incontinence	A: Arrhythmias	A: Arrhythmias
M: Miosis	T: Tachycardia	S: Slurred speech
B: Bronchorrhea, Bronchospasm	C: Cramps	H: Headache
B: Bradycardia	H: Hypertension	C: Confusion
E: Emesis		A: Ataxia
L: Lacrimation		T: Tremors
S: Secretions increased Salivation, Sweating		**[Late effects: ARC CC]**
		A: Areflexia
		R: Respiratory depression
		C: Circulatory depression
		C: Convulsions
		C: Coma

Management of acute poisoning

Diagnosis: Diagnosis of organophosphate poisoning is usually based on four criteria as shown in Figure 2.

Table 1: Neurological manifestations in OPC poisoning (Based on time of occurrence and pathophysiology)

Type I paralysis: Acute paralysis	*Type II paralysis: Organophosphate intermediate syndrome*	*Type III paralysis: Organophosphate-induced delayed peripheral polyneuropathy*
Acute onset postexposure *Cause:* Inhibition of AChE enzyme (acute cholinergic crisis). *Symptoms:* Muscle fasciculation, cramps, respiratory depression, etc. (*as described above in acute poisoning*). *Management:* Atropine, oximes and supportive treatment (*as described in detail later in the treatment section*)	*Occurs after 1–4 days of exposure.* *Cause:* Prolonged inhibition of AChE enzyme (may be due to inadequate treatment). *Symptoms:* Weakness of the proximal limb muscles and neck flexors *(distal muscle group is spared)*. Cranial nerve palsies (III to VII and X) *Management:* Supportive. (Atropine/Oximes are ineffective) *Resolution:* in 1–3 weeks	*Occurs after a latent period of 2–4 weeks (delayed sequelae)* *Cause:* Nerve demyelination/ sensory-motor distal axonopathy following ingestion of large amounts of organophosphates. *Symptoms:* Weakness, ataxia and paresthesia of the *distal* limb muscles. *Management:* Supportive. (Atropine/Oximes are ineffective) *Resolution:* in 1–2 months only of the sensory symptoms (paralysis persists).

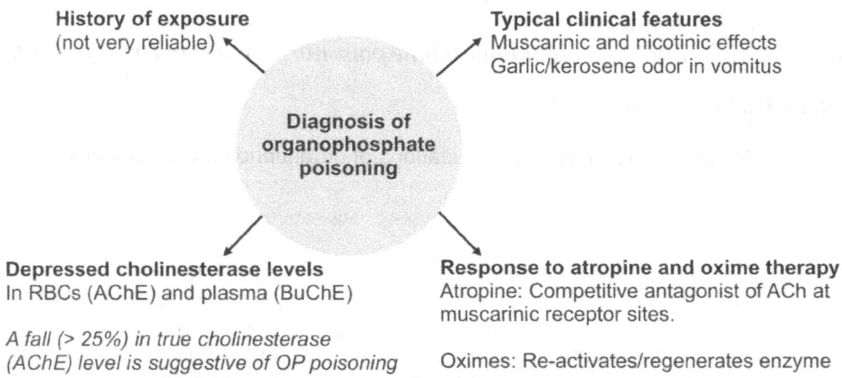

Fig. 2: Diagnosis of organophosphate poisoning

Note: The details of Type I and Type II cholinesterase enzymes are given in Table 2.

Table 2: Types and characteristics of cholinesterase enzyme

Cholinesterase enzyme (ChE)	*Type I ChE: True cholinesterase/ Acetylcholinesterase (AChE)*	*Type II ChE: Pseudocholinesterase/ Butyrylcholinesterase (BuChE)*
Produced in	RBCs	Liver
Found in	RBCs, gray matter, and motor end plates	Plasma, white matter, and visceral organs
Hydrolyses	Acetylcholine quickly	Butyrylcholine quickly
Levels after OP exposure	Decreased	Decreased
Indicator of poisoning	More reliable	Less reliable
Clinical manifestations	A fall in levels by $\geq$50%	--
Regeneration	Slow (1–3 months)	Early (few days to weeks)

Treatment

- Remove the victim from the site of exposure to fresh air
- Decontamination (wash the affected skin/eyes, and gastric lavage in case of ingestion)
- Airway protection (clear the airways of secretions periodically)
- Respiratory and cardiac monitoring—respiratory rate, arterial blood gas (ABG) analysis, ECG, etc.
- Supportive treatment—ventilatory and inotropic support
- Benzodiazepines for controlling convulsions
- *Toxin specific measures*:
  1. *Anticholinergics*: Administration of atropine*
  2. *Cholinesterase reactivators*: Administration of oximes such as pralidoxime (also known as 2-PAM or 2-pyridine aldoxime methylchloride), diacetylmonoxime (DAM), obidoxime, etc.

  **Atropine together with oximes is the most effective therapy in organophosphate poisoning.*
- *Atropine (Physiological antidote)*: It is a competitive antagonist of acetylcholine at muscarinic receptor sites. It reverses muscarinic effects and possibly CNS toxicity (does not reverse the skeletal muscle effects).
  - *Starting dose*: 2 mg IV bolus
  - *Subsequent doses*: 2–5 mg every 5–15 minutes until atropinization is achieved.

Note: Atropinization refers to increased heart rate (>100 beats/min), moderately dilated pupils, reduced bowel sounds, dry mouth and decrease in bronchial secretions.

- *Oximes (Specific antidote)*: Reactivates/regenerates the phosphorylated AChE. It reverses both nicotinic and muscarinic effects. Oximes are ineffective in cases of "Aging".

  Oxime therapy should be started as early as possible to prevent permanent binding of organophosphate to AChE and continued until adequate spontaneous ventilation is achieved.

  Dose is 1 g IV every 6–12 hours in adults (maximum dose 12 g/24 hours).

Postmortem appearances (Table 3)

Table 3: Postmortem findings in fatal OPC poisoning

External	*Internal*
• Froth from mouth and nostrils • Garlicky/Kerosene like odor from mouth	• Garlicky/Kerosene like odor in gastric contents • Pulmonary and cerebral edema • Congestion of organs

Notes: Garlicky odor is reported in Phosphorus, Organophosphates, Thallium and Arsenic poisoning (POTA). Kerosene/petrol like odor in OPC poisoning is due to the solvent used.

Medicolegal significance and circumstances of poisoning

- Organophosphates are most commonly used in form of field sprays and household chemicals.
- It is an occupational hazard for the farming community.
- Their easy availability and high toxicity makes them a preferred means of suicide.
- Accidental poisoning is reported mostly due to improper handling of the compounds.
- Homicides are rare owing to its disagreeable taste and odor, and due to the possibility of its detection after death even in the putrefied bodies (OPCs resist putrefaction).

- *Chemical warfare*: As nerve agents (e.g. Sarin gas)
- *Therapeutic uses*: (e.g. echothiophate in glaucoma)

Write a note on carbamate poisoning?

Mechanism of action

Carbamates like organophosphates (OPCs) are anticholinesterases that bind with the enzyme cholinesterase (ChE) and inhibit it by carbamylation (*OPCs cause phosphorylation of enzyme*). Likewise, accumulation of the ACh at the synapses causes overstimulation of muscarinic and nicotinic receptors. The inhibition is reversible as the enzyme is regenerated following spontaneous hydrolysis of carbamate (decarbamylation of enzyme) within 24–48 hours. Carbamates are not associated with "Aging".

Clinical manifestations

Clinical manifestations of carbamate poisoning are similar but less severe than organophosphate poisoning. Muscarinic symptoms **(Mnemonic *DUMBBELS*)** are most common, nicotinic symptoms **(Mnemonic *MATCH*)** are less frequent and CNS toxicity is rare.

Blood cholinesterase levels are not diagnostic as the levels return to normal within few hours.

Treatment

Atropine is the specific antidote. Role of oximes in treatment of carbamate poisoning is long debated. It is recommended that oximes are co-administered with atropine in all cases of carbamate poisoning *except* in carbaryl poisoning where it has been shown to do more harm than good. When oximes are co-administered with atropine, the effects are found to be positive or neutral.

Note: Mixed poisoning of OPCs and carbamates is not uncommon which may be difficult to differentiate clinically, further emphasizing on the need to co-administer atropine and oximes.

***It is a misconception that oximes are contraindicated in carbamate poisoning.*

Write a note on pyrethroid poisoning?

- Pyrethroids are synthetic analogs of naturally occurring pyrethrins present in the dried chrysanthemum (*Chrysanthemum cinerariifolium*) flower extract.
- Pyrethroids are important constituent of insect sprays and mosquito repellents.

Mechanism of action

Pyrethroids act primarily due to its affinity for membrane sodium and chloride channels. Nerve and muscle cells are the primary targets.

Pyrethroids have low systemic toxicity as these are poorly absorbed and rapidly metabolized.

Clinical manifestations

Clinical manifestations of acute poisoning:

- *Dermal exposure*: Tingling and burning sensation, numbness, erythema, pruritus and blistering.

- *Ocular exposure*: Irritation of eyes, itching, lacrimation, conjunctival and lid edema.
- *Inhalation*: Irritation of nasal and respiratory mucosa, sneezing, throat pain, wheezing, cough, dyspnea, chest pain, pneumonitis and pulmonary edema.
- *Ingestion*: Gastrointestinal irritation, nausea, vomiting, diarrhea and abdominal cramps.
- *Systemic toxicity*: Fatigue, dizziness, headache, fasciculations, tremors, and seizures. Hypotension, tachycardia, seizures and coma may occur at large doses. Convulsions and coma are life-threatening.

Cause of death

Respiratory failure.

Diagnosis

It is usually based on the history of exposure. Diagnostic difficulty is owed to its similarity with organophosphate poisoning. Blood cholinesterase levels are however, normal in Pyrethroid poisoning.

Management

- Remove the victim from the site of exposure to fresh air.
  - Decontamination (wash the affected skin/eyes, and gastric lavage in case of ingestion)
  - *No specific antidote is available for management of pyrethroid poisoning*
  - Symptomatic and supportive treatment
  - Benzodiazepines for controlling prolonged seizures.

**Atropine and oximes are not indicated in pyrethroids poisoning.*

Medicolegal significance/circumstances of poisoning

- Occupational exposure may occur through dermal contact and inhalation
- Unintentional/accidental exposure from household applications containing pyrethroids
- Intentional/suicidal intake of pyrethroids may occur due to its easy availability.

Describe in detail about aluminium phosphide toxicity including its mechanism of action, clinical manifestations, management, postmortem findings and medicolegal significance?

Aluminium phosphide is available in the form of greenish grey tablets (3 g each) or pellets (0.6 g each) for its use as a pesticide (grain preservative).

It is available in the market by names alphos, celphos, quickphos, phostoxin, etc.

Mechanism of toxicity

Metal phosphides release highly toxic phosphine gas (PH_3) when exposed to moisture or by the action of hydrochloric acid in the stomach.

$AlP + 3\,H_2O \rightarrow Al(OH)_3 + PH_3\uparrow$

$AlP + 3\,HCl \rightarrow AlCl_3 + PH_3\uparrow$

(3 g AlP tablet releases 1 g PH_3; 0.6 g AlP pellet releases 0.2 g PH_3)

Phosphine gas is rapidly absorbed on ingestion/inhalation. It blocks the enzyme cytochrome C oxidase, thus, inhibiting the mitochondrial oxidative phosphorylation. Mitochondrial cytochrome C oxidase inhibition causes cellular hypoxia and results in widespread organ damage (cytotoxic phosphine gas).

Clinical manifestations

- *Ingestion of AlP*: Nausea, vomiting, diarrhea, abdominal pain, restlessness, palpitation, pulmonary edema, cyanosis, hypotension, shock, ARDS (adult respiratory distress syndrome) and cardiac arrhythmias. Other effects include hepatitis, acute tubular necrosis, disseminated intravascular coagulation, metabolic acidosis and/or respiratory alkalosis. Phosphine gas may cause multiorgan failure/hepatic failure, renal failure, cardiac failure, clotting abnormalities, etc.
- *Inhalation of PH_3 gas*: Respiratory and gastrointestinal distress, headache, pulmonary edema, ARDS, cold and clammy sweats, tremors, convulsions, delirium, coma, congestive cardiac failure (CCF), arrhythmias, etc.

  Fatal dose: 1–3 tablets

  Fatal period: 1– 3 days

Diagnosis

The diagnosis is based on the detection of phosphine gas in breath/vomitus/gastric aspirate/tissues:

- Garlicky/decaying fish odor in breath/around the body

Note: Pure phosphine is odorless. The garlicky/decaying fish odor is due to the substituted phosphine and diphosphane (P_2H_4) gas.

- ECG changes include arrhythmias and heart blocks.
- Silver nitrate impregnated paper test: Filter paper impregnated with silver nitrate solution when exposed to breath/vomitus/gastric aspirate/minced tissues turns black as silver nitrate ($AgNO_3$) is reduced to Ag. On adding a drop of ammonium molybdate solution, black filter paper turns blue.
- Ammonium molybdate test: Appearance of canary yellow precipitate is confirmatory.
- Gas chromatography: is the most specific and sensitive method.

Management

- Gastric lavage and activated charcoal administration (1 g charcoal per kg body weight).
- No specific antidote is known. Intravenous magnesium sulfate is suggested as specific therapy.
  - *Magnesium sulfate* to correct hypomagnesemia and for effective management of arrhythmias.
  - Coconut oil can be an effective antidote in acute aluminium phosphide poisoning.
- Treatment is mostly symptomatic and supportive.
- Oxygen therapy/intubation and assisted ventilation to manage respiratory distress/ARDS.
- Sodium bicarbonate is administered to correct metabolic acidosis
- Intravenous fluids and appropriate vasopressors are given to treat shock.

Cause of death

Cardiac arrhythmias, metabolic acidosis and/or respiratory alkalosis, ARDS/multiorgan failure.

Postmortem appearances (Table 4)

Table 4: Postmortem findings in aluminium phosphide poisoning

External	Internal
• Garlicky/decaying fish odor from mouth • Blood mixed froth from mouth and nostrils.	• Froth in trachea • Garlicky/decaying fish odor in gastric contents. Presence of remnants of alphos tablets in stomach. Gastric distension with PH_3 gas, and gastrointestinal hemorrhages/congestion. • Pulmonary edema and hemorrhages in the interlobular areas and at the margins of the lungs • Brain is edematous; organs are congested.

Medicolegal significance/circumstances of poisoning

- AlP poisoning occurs mostly due to its suicidal ingestion or at times due to accidental ingestion of AlP or inhalation of phosphine gas.
- AlP is reportedly the most common cause of poisoning in parts of Northern India.

Write a note on zinc phosphide poisoning?

Zinc phosphides are used a rodenticide.

Mechanism of action: Release of phosphine gas when it comes in contact with moisture/acid. Toxicity is due to phosphine gas, similar to, and as described in AlP.

The rate of phosphine release and appearance of symptoms however, is comparatively slower than AlP.

Clinical manifestations

Garlicky/decaying fish odor in breath, abdominal pain, vomiting, diarrhea, metabolic acidosis, hypotension, shock, respiratory distress, convulsions, coma, etc.

Cause of death

Metabolic acidosis, pulmonary edema, ARDS/multiorgan failure.

Treatment

No specific antidote.

Gastric lavage followed by symptomatic and supportive therapy similar to that mentioned in AlP poisoning.

Write a note on paraquat poisoning?

Paraquat is an herbicide with ammonia like odor.

Clinical manifestations

- *Mild poisoning (consumption of <20 mg paraquat ion/kg of body weight)*: Mild gastrointestinal symptoms.
- *Moderate-to-severe poisoning (consumption of 20–40 mg paraquat ion/kg of body weight)*: Vomiting, pain abdomen, oral and throat burns/ulcers, pulmonary fibrosis, breathing difficulty, seizures, etc.

- *Acute fulminant poisonings (consumption of >40 mg of paraquat ion/kg of body weight)*: Organs like kidney, liver and the heart are affected, resulting in multiple organ (cardiac, respiratory, renal, hepatic, adrenal, pancreatic, and neurological) failure.

Complication

Lungs are often involved.

Progressive pulmonary fibrosis (***Paraquat lung***) is a common complication.

Fatal dose

30–50 mg/kg body weight

Cause of death

Respiratory or multiorgan failure.

Treatment

- Supportive and symptomatic treatment.
- Gastrointestinal decontamination is attempted in patients who present early following ingestion of paraquat.
- *Oxygen therapy may precipitate pulmonary fibrosis and, hence, given judiciously.*

Drug Dependence and Drug Abuse

CHAPTER 19

Define drug dependence. What are its various types? Mention the criteria for diagnosis of dependence syndrome?

The terms "drug addiction" and "drug habituation" were replaced by the term "drug dependence" globally on the suggestions made by the WHO in 1964. In ICD-10 diagnostic guidelines, the term "dependence syndrome" is used for "drug dependence".

Drug dependence

- Drug dependence principally refers to *"a state in which the individual has a need for repeated doses of the drug to feel good or to avoid feeling bad"*. Broadly, dependence comprises of both physical and psychological components.
- Drug dependence is defined as *"a state, psychic and sometimes also physical resulting from the interaction between a living organism and a drug, characterized by behavioral and other responses that always include a compulsion to take the drug on a continuous or periodic basis in order to experience its psychic effects, and sometimes to avoid the discomfort of its absence"*.

Dependence syndrome

Dependence syndrome refers to a strong desire to take psychoactive drugs, alcohol, or tobacco.

- *ICD-10 definition*: *"A cluster of physiological, behavioral, and cognitive phenomena in which the use of a substance or a class of substances takes on a much higher priority for a given individual than other behaviors that once had greater value"*.

Types of dependence

- *Psychological or psychic dependence*: Compulsive use of drugs for individual satisfaction. An individual believes that the state of well-being is associated with use of a particular substance. No withdrawal symptoms appear on cessation, e.g. tea, coffee, tobacco, lysergic acid diethylamide (LSD), etc.
- *Physical or Physiological dependence*: It is associated with altered physiological state. Withdrawal symptoms appear on cessation of drug.

WHO Expert Committee on Drug Dependence (ECDD) identifies different types of dependence based on the group of drugs producing it. These are:

- Amphetamine type
- Barbiturate/sedative type

- Cocaine type
- Cannabis type
- Morphine type
- Hallucinogen type
- Ethanol type
- Tobacco type
- Caffeine type.

Diagnostic guidelines of dependence syndrome (ICD-10 diagnostic guidelines)

A positive diagnosis of dependence should usually be made only if at least three of the following six criteria are present together at some time during the previous year:

1. Compulsive desire to take the substance (craving)
2. Difficulties in controlling substance taking behavior
3. Characteristic *withdrawal syndrome* on cessation of the substance
4. Development of *tolerance*
5. Progressive neglect of alternative pleasures or interests
6. Persistent use despite of the awareness about associated harmful consequences.

Write briefly on tolerance and withdrawal syndrome?

Tolerance

Increased doses are required in order to achieve effects originally produced by lower doses. Such individuals may tolerate very high doses (harmful/fatal enough for others).

Note: Cross tolerance refers to tolerance for pharmacologically related drugs, e.g. alcoholics are tolerant to barbiturates.

Withdrawal syndrome

Group of symptoms of variable clustering and severity occurring on absolute or relative withdrawal of a substance after its repeated and usually prolonged use.

Mention the difference between drug habituation and drug addiction?

Addiction and habituation are produced by the repeated use of a drug to cause dependence. Drug dependence is inclusive of the terms "drug addiction" and "drug habituation" (Table 1).

Table 1: Differences between drug addiction and habituation

	*Drug addiction**	*Drug habituation*
Dependence	Physical and psychological	Only psychological
Compulsive desire	Yes	No
Desire to increase dose	Yes	No
Withdrawal symptoms	Yes (specific for the drug)	None or mild
Tolerance	Yes	No
Social issues	Yes	No
Individual harm	Yes	No/May be
Substances/Agents	Cocaine, morphine, alcohol	Caffeine, tobacco

*Addiction is not an accepted scientific term. In lay terms, it refers to severe dependence.
Addiction evolves through the stages; psychological dependence, physical dependence and tolerance.

Write a note on drug abuse versus drug maladministration?

- *Drug abuse* (misuse or nonmedical use of drugs) refers to *intentional* use of excessive doses of prescribed drugs, or use of therapeutic doses for reasons other than what the drug was prescribed for. Drug abuse is, thus, defined as *"persistent or sporadic excessive drug use inconsistent with or unrelated to acceptable medical practice"*. Drug abuse may or may not cause dependence. Similarly, all dependence producing drugs are not abused (e.g. caffeine).
  - DSM-IV-TR makes no reference of the term "drug abuse", but mentions "substance abuse".

Note: Drug dependence resulting from acceptable medicinal use of dependence producing drugs does not amount to drug abuse.

- *Drug maladministration* refers to *unintentional* (accidental) use of drugs that includes inappropriate/indiscriminate prescribing of drugs or prescription errors.

Write a note on drug carriers and its variants. Differentiate between body packers and body stuffers? What is body packer syndrome?

Drug carriers are individuals involved in trafficking/smuggling of illicit substances/drugs by concealing these in the body (intracorporeal concealment). It was first reported in 1970s.

The carriers are commonly used for smuggling of cocaine (cocaine body packers), or heroin (heroin body packers). Hashish, LSD, ecstasy, etc. are rarely transported through the carriers.

Categories/variants of drug carriers

Categories/variants of drug carriers are described in Table 2.

Table 2: Categories/variants of drug carriers

1. Body *packers*	• Also called "internal carriers", "swallowers", "mules", or "couriers" • Carrier who *swallows packets* of illicit drug in GI tract for smuggling
2. Body pushers	Carrier who *hides drug containers* in body cavities (rectum, vagina, etc.)
3. Body *stuffers*	• Also called "mini packers" or "quick swallowers". • Usually keep pellets in cheek pouch, and swallows these when confronted by law enforcing authorities to evade detection or arrest.

The variant "body pushers" is often included in "body packers" since the purpose of carrying the illicit drugs is the same (smuggling across international borders). They differ in the site of hiding of the illicit drug and the size of the packages (larger in body pushers). Mouth, esophagus, ear and foreskin are the other sites reported for hiding illicit drugs. The details of body packers and body stuffers are described in Table 3.

Packages

Packages are known as bolos, pellets, condoms, finger stalls, etc. The packets are multilayered. The inner layer pouching the compressed drug is made of balloons, condoms, finger stalls or plastic bags (tied or heat-sealed at one end), and is well-covered with layers of latex/polythene. Aluminium foil, plastic, carbon paper, toilet/filter paper is often added as intermediary layers. The packages are either handmade/manually wrapped (variable shape and size) or produced mechanically (uniform morphology). The packets meant to be ingested are round/oval and smaller (3–6 cm long, 1–2 cm diameter, each containing 8–12 g of drug) while those to be inserted in body cavities are oval and larger (length up to 15 cm).

Table 3: Characteristic differentiating features of body packers and body stuffers

	Body packers	*Body stuffers*
Slang terms (synonyms)	"internal carriers", "swallowers", "mules", and "couriers"	"Mini packers" and "Quick swallowers"
Offender	Specifically hired for smuggling	Street dealer or abuser himself
Prior training	Offender is well trained	None usually
Timing of intake	Premeditated and well in advance	Swallows on the verge of arrest
Purpose/Intention	Trafficking across international borders	To evade detection/arrest in an unexpected encounter with police
Size of packets	Larger (3–6 cm x 1–2 cm)	Smaller (pellets of 1 cm diameter)
Number of packets	50–100 packets of 8–12 g each	Fewer in number
Quantity of drug	Large amount (around 1 kg)	Smaller amounts
Purity of drug	Typically carry high purity drugs	Lower purity
Quality of packing	Good, packets are well-prepared	Poorly wrapped pouches or pellets
Medications	Common (antimotility drugs)	Rare
Risk of intoxication	Less	More (since packaging is poor)
Radiography	Detection is relatively easier	More difficult (smaller size and dose)
Management	Whole bowel irrigation (WBI)	Laxatives alone may help
Surgical removal	May be required	Not usually
Advantage	Large amounts are transported	Detection is difficult

Procedure

Body packers swallow the packets containing drugs and engage in drug trafficking. Antimotility drugs (loperamide or diphenoxylate, etc.) are taken to reduce bowel movements. On arrival at the destination, mild laxatives or enemas are used for retrieval of the packets in the feces. The packets are sometimes vomited out.

Complications

Drug intoxication, intestinal obstruction, perforation, peritonitis, etc.

Site of obstruction is usually the pylorus, and rarely ileocecal valve.

Medicolegal investigations

Drug screening and radiography.

Radiography

Radiological investigations are primarily aimed to identify the carrier (concealed packets), and also report the exact location and number of packets. X-ray is most commonly employed for initial screening (packets appear as multiple round/oval shadows similar to feces in density), and noncontrast CT is considered as gold standard for diagnosis of both body packers and stuffers. Besides, the exact number and location, the CT can also identify the ruptured packets which are smaller, irregular, and of different density than the others.

The following radiological signs are typically useful in identification of drug carriers:

- *"Tic-tac sign"*: Multiple uniform round/oval densities in the GI lumen (very common)
- *"Rosette sign"*: Due to air trapped in the twisted end of a package tied with bindings
- *"Double condom sign"*: Due to air trapped between layers, that appears as a halo/crescent. Also appreciated in body stuffers. Rosette and double condom sign are better appreciated in the CT scans.
- *"Parallelism sign"*: Due to parallel aligned packets in the GI lumen (not common).

Body packer syndrome

Body packer syndromes are clinical manifestations of the drug (usually cocaine or heroin) intoxication following the rupture or leakage of the packets. Rupture may be caused due to the direct action of gastric acid on the wraps, while leakage occurs due to diffusion of drugs through the semipermeable wrap, or due to poor quality of packing causing intoxication.

Management

- Whole bowel irrigation with polyethylene glycol (PEG) is the treatment of choice.
- Symptomatic and specific treatment for cocaine/heroin intoxication should continue.
- Surgical intervention is required in cases of intestinal obstruction, perforation, severe intoxication, etc.

Cause of death

Acute drug intoxication, esophageal/bowel perforation and peritonitis.

What is drug-facilitated sexual assault (DFSA)? Mention about "date rape" and enumerate some "date rape drugs"?

Drug-facilitated sexual assault (DFSA) or "predator rape" refers to sexual assault on an incapacitated person who is under the influence of any mind-altering substances such as alcohol or other date rape drugs.

- Alcohol-facilitated sexual assaults are the most common form of DFSA worldwide.
- "Date rape" refers to sexual assault carried out by an acquaintance during/following a "date" (social meeting of couples). The assault may be forced on a well-conscious nonconsenting victim or the victim is incapacitated by alcohol or drugs (date rape drugs) to carry out DFSA. The mind-altering substances may be consumed voluntary or administered by the perpetrator.
- Date rape is a variant of "acquaintance rape".

"Date rape drug" or *"Predator drug"* refers to any substance that incapacitates a person and makes her vulnerable to DFSA. Date rape drugs are often introduced in the drinks of the unsuspecting victim so that the victim is unable to give a reasoned consent or resist the sexual advances. Some of the common date rape drugs/substances apart from *alcohol* are:

- *Micky Finn/Knock out drops* (solution of alcohol and chloral hydrate)
- *Flunitrazepam (Rohypnol)* also known as circles, forget pill, R-2, roach, rope, etc.
- *GHB (gamma-hydroxybutyric acid)* also known as bedtime scoop, easy lay, G, G-juice, energy drink, grievous bodily harm (GBH), liquid ecstasy, liquid X, etc.
- *Ketamine* also known as black hole, bump, green, purple, jet, kit kat, K, special K, K-hole, psychedelic heroin, super acid, etc.
- *Club drugs/rave drugs/party drugs such as "Ecstasy" (MDMA).*

CHAPTER 20 Food Poisoning

Write a short note on food poisoning and its types.

Food poisoning (foodborne illness) is an illness of infectious or toxic nature following consumption of contaminated food or drinks. Food may be contaminated by fungi, bacteria, viruses, toxins present in plants and animals, and chemicals, etc. (Flowchart 1).

Nausea, vomiting and diarrhea are the common clinical manifestations.

Treatment includes oral rehydration solutions and antibiotics specific for causative bacteria.

Note: "Food allergies" (e.g. hypersensitivity following ingestion of milk, eggs, sea food, etc.) are generally not included as "food poisoning".

Flowchart 1: Types of food poisoning

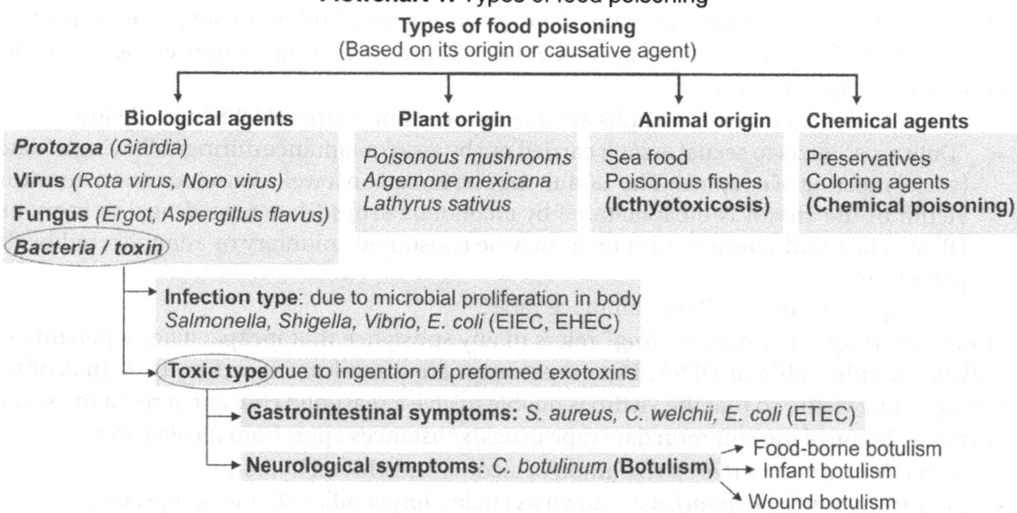

Write a short note on botulism/allantiasis.

Botulism: A potentially fatal illness caused by botulinum toxin (exotoxin/neurotoxin).

Causative organism: *Clostridium botulinum* (a gram positive, spore forming anaerobic bacilli).

Types

- *Food-borne botulism*: Consumption of food contaminated with *preformed toxin.*
- *Infant botulism (Intestinal botulism)*: Consumption of *botulinum spores* which grows in intestine and release exotoxin. (Ingestion of spores does not cause botulism in adults.)
- *Wound botulism*: Release of toxin in wounds infested with *botulinum spores.*
- *Inhalation botulism*: Release of *toxins* in aerosols intentionally (e.g. bioterrorism) or accidentally (e.g. in laboratories).

Source: Inadequately processed food, canned/tinned meat products (sausages, etc.), fish, fruits, vegetables and ready-to-eat foods are potential sources for foodborne botulism.

Spore-contaminated honey has been implicated in infant botulism.

Transmission

Clostridium botulinum spores are heat-resistant and exist widely around us. In the absence of oxygen they germinate, grow and release powerful exotoxins.

Exotoxins

There are seven immunologically distinct types of botulinum toxins (A to G).

- Types A, B, E and rarely F are associated with human botulism (Type A is most lethal)
- Types C, D and E are responsible for intoxication in land and aquatic animals.

Mechanism of action

Botulinum toxin is a neurotoxin that acts by presynaptic binding to cholinergic nerve fibers. The toxin inhibits the release of acetylcholine from nerve terminals causing flaccid paralysis.

Incubation period

½ to 1½ days (12–36 hours).

Lethal dose

Botulinum toxins are the most lethal toxin. Lethal dose in humans is 0.001 μg/kg.

Clinical manifestations

- *Food-borne botulism*: Marked fatigue, weakness, blurring of vision (diplopia), dryness of mouth, dysphonia (difficulty in speaking), dysphagia (difficulty in swallowing), vomiting, diarrhea, distension of abdomen may occur. The weakness progresses to muscles of neck and arms, respiratory muscles and muscles of the lower body, (descending motor paralysis) and difficulty in breathing (Box 1 and 2).

  **Characteristic symptoms are due to bulbar palsy and symmetric descending motor paralysis.*

  No fever *No loss of consciousness*
- *Wound botulism and inhalation botulism*: Symptoms are similar to the foodborne botulism, but may take relatively longer time to appear.
- *Infant botulism*: Constipation, poor feeding, diminished/altered cry, neck muscle weakness and loss of head control.

Box 1: Clinical manifestations of Botulism; **Mnemonic:** ***8 Ds***

- **D**iplopia
- **D**ry mouth
- **D**ysphonia
- **D**ysphagia
- **D**iarrhea
- **D**istended abdomen
- **D**escending motor paralysis
- **D**ifficulty in breathing.

Box 2: Characteristic features of Botulism; **Mnemonic:** ***4Bs***

- **B**ulbar palsy
- **B**ilateral descending motor paralysis
- **B**reathing difficulty
- **B**iological warfare (Bioterrorism)

Cause of death

Respiratory muscle paralysis leading to respiratory failure.

Diagnosis

Based on history of consumption of contaminated food (honey in infants) and clinical examination. Stool culture for presence of *Clostridium botulinum*, and presence of toxin in serum, stool or food are confirmatory.

Differential diagnosis

Guillain-Barré syndrome, Myasthenia gravis.

Treatment

- Symptomatic and supportive treatment especially respiratory care.
- *Specific treatment*: Trivalent antitoxin (A, B, and E) should be administered at the earliest.
- *Infant botulism*: Botulism immune globulin (BIG) is administered (it neutralizes types A and B botulinum toxins).
- *Wound botulism*: Antibiotics (antibiotics are not given in other variants of botulism).
- *Inhalation/Contact botulism*: Immediate decontamination (bathing with soap and water).

Prevention

- Boiling/pressure cooking destroys botulinum toxins (spores are heat-resistant; toxins are not)
- Avoid feeding honey to the infants.

Medicolegal aspects

- Accidental poisonings due to consumption of contaminated food
- Botulism as an agent of biological warfare/bioterrorism.
- Mild and transient adverse effects in application of Botox® (Botulinum toxin type A) in dermocosmetology practice.

Write a short note on poisoning with mushrooms.

Mushroom poisoning: Occurs due to consumption of poisonous mushrooms (Table 1).

Table 1: Active principles and action of poisonous mushrooms

Poisonous mushroom	Active principles	Action
Amanita muscaria (Fly agaric)	Muscarine	Stimulates postganglionic cholinergic fibers
Amanita phalloides (Death cap)	Phalloidin, α-amanitin	Inhibit cellular protein synthesis *(Phalloides syndrome)*

Symptoms

Symptoms vary in different varieties (onset is early in muscarine and delayed in amanitin poisoning). In general, symptoms can be described as:

- *Irritant symptoms*: Abdominal pain, throat irritation, nausea, vomiting, and diarrhea
- *Neurotic symptoms*: Headache, giddiness, delirium, visual disturbances, diplopia, excessive salivation, sweating, cramps, bradycardia, difficulty in breathing, convulsions, coma, and death.
- *Hepatic and renal toxicity* may occur in 3–6 days (in amanitin/amatoxin poisoning).

Fatal dose
1–2 mushrooms (depends on species)

Fatal period
1 day (24 hours)

Treatment

- Decontamination and administration of activated charcoal
- Supportive treatment especially respiratory care, rehydration with fluid therapy
- *Specific treatment for muscarine poisoning*: *Intravenous atropine sulfate.*
- *Specific treatment for phalloidin poisoning: Antiphalloidin antibodies.*
- Benzyl penicillin, cimetidine and *N*-acetylcysteine in amatoxin poisoning.
- *Symptomatic treatment*: Diazepam for convulsions, hemodialysis in renal toxicity and liver transplantation for hepatic failure.

Write a short note on "Ptomaines".

Ptomaines

Ptomaines are alkaloids formed as a byproduct of bacterial decomposition of proteins.

- Ptomaines that are formed in dead tissues rich in protein are referred as *"cadaveric alkaloids"*.
- Similarly, ptomaines formed in living cells are called *"leukomaines"*.
  - "Neurine" and "mydalein" are the most toxic ptomaines.
  - Ptomaine poisoning was often related to consumption of canned meat products, sausages, etc.
  - Phrase "ptomaine poisoning" is rarely used now as the actual cause of food poisoning attributed to "ptomaines" was observed to be bacterial in origin.

Write a short note on "Lathyrism".

Lathyrism

Lathyrism, also referred to as "*Neurolathyrism*" is a crippling disease that occurs due to excessive consumption of *Lathyrus sativus* (Kesari dal, Grass pea) over 3–6 months. The disease is prevalent in the lower socioeconomic settings and is reported from India, Nepal, Bangladesh, and Ethiopia, etc. The condition is more common in men, and mostly affects younger people.

Mechanism of toxicity
The exact mechanism is unclear. However, neurotoxicity is believed to be due to β-N-oxalylamino-L-alanine (BOAA), also known as β-N-oxalyl-L-α,β-diaminopropionic acid (ODAP).

Clinical manifestations
Neurolathyrism" is characterized by *progressive spastic paraplegia*.

Its progression is described in four stages:

1. *Stage I (No stick stage)*: Muscle spasms and weakness of the lower limbs. Painful knee and ankle movements. Difficulty in sitting down and getting up.
2. *Stage II (One stick stage)*: Marked flexion of the knee and inversion of foot with a tendency to walk on toes (spastic gait and tip toe walking).
3. *Stage III (Two stick stage)*: Further deterioration. Can walk only with crutches/sticks.
4. *Stage IV (Crawler stage)*: Knee is completely flexed. Inability to walk/bedridden.

Thus, the gait becomes progressively unsteady due to muscular spasticity and paraplegia of lower extremities. Patient is crippled and is confined to bed. Sensation and sphincters are spared. Mind remains clear, and death is rare.

Management

No specific treatment. Once kesari dal is removed from the daily diet, the symptoms cease to progress. Physiotherapy is helpful.

Prevention

Removal of the toxin by steeping the pulse in hot water and parboiling it.

Restricted use of kesari dal in daily diet (<25% of the diet), and Vitamin C prophylaxis.

Note: Osteolathyrism (Odoratism) affects bones and connecting tissues due to ingestion of Lathyrus odoratus seeds (Sweet peas); the toxin responsible is β-aminopropionitrile.

Write a note on medicolegal aspects of food poisoning.

- *Accidental poisonings* commonly occurs following consumption of contaminated food/ poisonous mushrooms.
- *Adulteration* of pulses (with *L. sativus*) and mustard oil (with *A. mexicana*), etc. cause serious illnesses (Table 2).

Table 2: Common adulterants, their active principles and the resulting illnesses

Adulterant	*Active principles*	*Illness*
Lathyrus sativus (Kesari Dal)	BOAA (β-N-oxalyl amino alanine) *in seeds*	Neurolathyrism
Argemone mexicana	Sanguinarine and dihydrosanguinarine in *oil*	Epidemic dropsy

- *Chemical poisoning due to additives and preservatives*: MSG (Monosodium glutamate) has been banned in some parts of world due to its deleterious health effects.
- *Criminal liability*: Adulteration of food or drink intended for sale (Section 272 IPC) and sale of noxious food or drink is a criminal offence (Section 273 IPC).
- *Biological warfare/Bioterrorism*: Botulism is a potential weapon of mass destruction.
- *Notifying public health authorities*: All food poisoning cases are to be reported to public health officer (exception to privileged communications)
- *Preservation*: Food samples are to be preserved, sealed and sent to laboratories for analysis.
- *Medical negligence issues*: For adverse effects in Botox® application in cosmetology practice.

CHAPTER 21

Common Household Poisons

Enumerate the various products used in the households including the common therapeutic agents that can cause poisoning. Mention their toxic ingredients, specific treatment and characteristic features in poisonings with these agents?

Various products used in the households including the common therapeutic agents that can cause poisoning have been described in Table 1.

Table 1: Various household products and their toxic ingredients, specific treatment and characteristic features

Product	Toxic ingredient	Specific treatment	Remarks
Antifreeze	Ethylene glycol (Metabolites: Oxalic acid, glycolic acid)	Ethanol, fomepizole, hemodialysis,**	Renal failure, hypocalcemia, Ca oxalate crystals in urine
Nail polish remover	Acetone, ethyl acetate	Oxygen therapy methylene blue,**	Inhalation abuse Methemoglobinemia Chronic CNS toxicity
Deodorants, air fresheners	Butane, propane, fluorocarbons, etc.	**	Inhalation abuse
Deodorants, air fresheners	Potassium permanganate	**, Methylene blue	Corrosive action, Methemoglobinemia
Paint thinner	Toluene, methylene chloride, methanol	**	Inhalation abuse Aspiration pneumonitis
Furniture polish	Turpentine, petroleum hydrocarbons	Oxygen therapy,**	Inhalation abuse Aspiration pneumonitis
Detergents	Corrosive agents	**	Corrosive action (mild)
Drain cleaners	Sodium hydroxide	**	Corrosive base toxicity
Bleaching powder	Calcium hypochlorite (Release chlorine and chloramine)	**	• Ingestion: Corrosive • Inhalation: Irritant
Baking powder	Sodium bicarbonate, tartaric acid	**, Hemodialysis	Metabolic alkalosis
Baking soda	Sodium bicarbonate	**	Metabolic alkalosis
Mothballs	Paradichlorobenzene, naphthalene, camphor	Methylene blue Packed RBCs,**	Methemoglobinemia, acute intravascular hemolysis—Anemia
Fireworks, matchstick head	Potassium chlorate, antimony (III) sulfide	Methylene blue hemodialysis	Methemoglobinemia, DIC, nephrotoxicity

Contd...

Contd...

Product	Toxic ingredient	Specific treatment	Remarks
Ants and Roach killer powder	Boric acid, borax pesticides (OPC/carbamate/pyrethroids)	Hemodialysis Atropine,**	Nephrotoxicity, neurotoxicity
• Mosquito repellents • Odomos cream	• Pyrethroids (kerosene solvent) • N, N-diethyl-benzamide	** **	Serious complications: Seizures, coma Dermatitis
Chalk (Lakshmanrekha)	Cypermethrin (pyrethroids)	**	Convulsions (rarely)
Rat poison	Metal phosphides, anticoagulants (warfarin, difethialone)	Mg sulfate Vitamin K,**	Multiple organ failure, internal bleeding liver and kidney damage
Pesticides	OPC, carbamates, etc.	See Chapter 18 on Agrochemicals	
Ink remover	Oxalic acid	See Chapter 5 on Corrosives	
Bleaching agents (Hair bleach)	Hydrogen peroxide (oxygen gas formation)	Airway management, Gastric tube	Corrosive action, oxygen embolization, abdominal bloating
Hair dye	Paraphenylenediamine (PPD)	** Dialysis	Cervicofascial edema, rhabdomyolysis, ARF
Ink, shoe polish	Aniline dye derivatives	Methylene blue,**	Methemoglobinemia
Paint remover	Alcohols, formic acid, naptha, and xylene,	**	Breathing difficulty, convulsions, coma
Thermometer spills	Elemental mercury	**	Toxicity unlikely (in oral intake) Vapors are toxic
Parad tablet	Mercury	Chelation, **	Acute renal failure
Dishwashing liquid/detergents	Sodium lauryl sulfate, sodium laureth sulfate, sodium polyphosphates, propylene glycol	**	Liver and kidney damage
Shampoo	Ammonium chloride, ammonium and sodium lauryl sulfate, sodium laureth sulfate	**	--
Button batteries	Mercuric oxide, nickel, cadmium, silver	Chelation,**	Cardiovascular collapse
Kerosene/Petrol			Discussed in detail in this chapter.
Common therapeutic agents:			
Antitussives/ Cough remedies	Dextromethorphan/Codeine/ Promethazine	Naloxone,**	Substance abuse, neurobehavioral disorders
Iron tonics/capsules	Iron salts	Chelation,**	Metabolic acidosis, hepatic failure
Sleeping pills	Benzodiazepines, Barbiturates (less often)	Flumazenil, **	Substance dependence, tolerance
Analgesics	Salicylates, aspirin	**	Respiratory alkalosis, metabolic acidosis
Analgesic and antipyretic	Acetaminophen, paracetamol	**, N-acetyl cysteine (NAC)	Hepatic necrosis, ARF

Contd...

Contd...

Product	Toxic ingredient	Specific treatment	Remarks
Antiseptics/ disinfectants (Dettol, Savlon)	Chloroxylenol, chlorhexidine gluconate, cetrimide	Airway management,**	Corrosion, aspiration, ARDS, CNS depression
Antiseptic powder	Boric acid	Hemodialysis,**	Nephrotoxicity
Antiseptic/ antifungal agents	Potassium permanganate	**, Methylene blue	Corrosive action, methemoglobinemia

Abbreviations: OPC, organophosphorous compound; ARF, acute respiratory failure; ARDS, acute respiratory distress syndrome; CNS, central nervous system

**Treatment is symptomatic. Gastric lavage is done whenever indicated.

Write a note on kerosene poisoning.

Mechanism of toxicity (pulmonary toxicity)

Kerosene vapors cause interstitial inflammation, intra-alveolar edema, bronchial necrosis, and *chemical pneumonitis.* Kerosene alters the surface tension of the alveolar membranes resulting in atelectasis and emphysema.

On ingestion, it has an irritant effect locally and causes respiratory depression and neurotoxicity on absorption.

Clinical manifestations

- Typical odor of kerosene in the breath
- Nausea, vomiting, epigastric pain, rarely gastrointestinal hemorrhages
- Chocking, coughing, dyspnea, crepitation, bronchopneumonia
- Headache, dizziness, ataxia, restlessness, pupils are constricted initially, and dilated in later stages.
- *In later stages*: Seizures, intravascular hemolysis, acute renal failure, cardiac arrhythmias, etc.

Complication

Aspiration pneumonitis

Fatal period

12–24 hours

Fatal dose

30–50 ml

Investigation

X-ray chest shows perihilar mottled opacities especially in the lower lobes.

Management

Shift the patient away from contamination.

- *Dermal/Ocular exposure*: Wash the affected part with soap and water.
- *Inhalation/Ingestion*: Airway management is the mainstay of treatment. Oxygen therapy.

In case of severe respiratory distress, early intubation and mechanical ventilation is attempted.

***Gastric lavage: Contraindicated due to the risk of aspiration (attempted only after intubation).**
***Antibiotic prophylaxis has limited role in the management of bronchopneumonia.**

Cause of death

Acute lung injury, respiratory failure

Medicolegal significance/circumstances of kerosene poisoning

- The most common route of poisoning is by ingestion, second most common being inhalation.
- Accidental poisoning is common in the pediatric age group.
- Suicidal poisoning in adults is rare, but not uncommon.
- Suicidal IV administration of kerosene has also been reported.
- Kerosene is not considered as a homicidal agent because of its peculiar odor.

CHAPTER 22

Poison Information Center

Write a short note on poison information center (PIC).

As per the WHO document, "*A poison center is a specialized unit that advises on, and assists with, the prevention, diagnosis and management of poisoning*". Poison centers at the least provide information services, and may have a toxicology laboratory and/or a clinical treatment unit associated with it.

Poison information center (PIC) is a specialized unit that provides round the clock information on early diagnosis, prevention, and management of poisoning, in principle to the whole community.

Objectives of PIC

(**Mnemonic:** ***PIC*** for **P**revention, **I**nformation and **C**ontrol)

- Provide prompt toxicological information and advice to individuals and healthcare providers.
- Reduce the cost of health care management
- Toxicovigilance activities and prevention of poisoning, recurrences, etc.
- Active research and provide training to health care professionals and community
- Awareness programs for different stakeholders, NGOs. etc.

Setting up of a PIC

- *Location*: Preferably near the emergency (Area around 1,000–1,500 square feet)
- *Staff requirements*: Director, medical toxicologist, poison information specialist, administrative and support staff.
- *Infrastructure*: Rooms with basic amenities for the director and the staff, office, library, computer room with databases for information services, and telephone facility for answering the calls/answering services.
- *Databases*: INTOX (WHO), POISINDEX (USA)
- *Timing*: Round the clock (24 × 7) services for all kinds of poisoning affecting all ages.

Functions of PIC

- *Information provider* (most important function) on toxicological aspects throughout the year
- *Toxicovigilance* and alerting the appropriate authorities for prevention of poisoning
- *Monitoring* the adverse effects of drugs, and in handling problems of substance abuse.

- *Research, education and training* aimed at the prevention and treatment of poisoning
- *Disaster preparedness*: Contingency planning and response to chemical incidents/disasters.

**Promptness, reliability, documentation and confidentiality are vital in functioning of a PIC.*

Operative procedure

Poison information center provides prompt information on poisons/poisoning through personal/telephonic enquiries, e-mails, post, etc. based on the well-recognized databases. Gather enquirer's demographics, followed by particulars of the victim, history of poisoning which includes name of substance/product, route of contact, quantity or strength, time since exposure, patient condition, health status, medication history, and allergy. Database is searched for appropriate resource and desired information. The first-aid management and/or treatment guidelines are transmitted to the enquirer. Access the progress; provide information on further referral, and any additional recommendation. Follow up the case until resolved. Information from the time of the first contact/call to the final outcome is noted which is periodically analyzed for quality assurance.

Poison information centers in India

The first PIC was established at All India Institute of Medical Sciences (AIIMS), New Delhi (1995) as National Poisons Information Center. Some of the other centers are located at Ahmedabad, Chennai and AIMS, Kochi.

CHAPTER 23

Problem Based Questions

1. A 45-year-old male during his job as a laboratory technician for the last 10 years has been exposed to concentrated vapors and spillage of chemicals. Lately he has complaints of anorexia, weakness, headache, muscle aches, and dark urine.

   (2 + 2 + 2 + 2 marks)

   a. What can be the probable diagnosis?
   b. Give reasons for your diagnosis.
   c. What is the probable cause of dark urine in this case?
   d. What other manifestations do you expect in this case?

2. A 50-year-old farmer presents to you in the emergency room with complaints of recurrent convulsive episodes. The patient has never had convulsions in the past. The patient is alert and conscious. Relatives told that the patient had complained of headache for which he had taken some herbal medicine a couple of hours back. Backward arching of the body is evident during the convulsive episode; otherwise, the muscles are in relaxed state.

   (2 + 2 + 2 + 2 marks)

   a. What is your likely diagnosis?
   b. What was the possible differential diagnosis that you arrived at in this case?
   c. Give reasons for your diagnosis.
   d. How will you manage this case?

3. A middle-aged worker suddenly collapsed during cleaning a septic tank. He was brought dead to casualty and autopsy was performed. Fine froth was present at the mouth and nostrils with a characteristic offensive odor appreciable at autopsy. Greenish discoloration of the skin, airways, viscera especially of the lungs and the brain surface was also observed.

   (2 + 2 + 2 + 2 marks)

   a. What is the possible diagnosis? Give reasons?
   b. What is the possible cause of death in this case?
   c. How will you confirm the diagnosis?
   d. What antidote should be administered if the patient had survived?

4. A young child has swallowed some liquid while playing in his house. He is brought to emergency initially with complaints of epigastric pain and vomiting followed by breathlessness. X-ray chest shows perihilar mottled opacities in the lower lobes bilaterally.

Gastric lavage was done promptly but the condition of the child worsened rapidly. Relatives claim medical negligence alleging lack of care and skill on part of the casualty medical officer.

(2 + 2 + 2 + 2 marks)

a. What is the possible diagnosis?
b. Give reasons for your diagnosis?
c. How will you effectively manage this case?
d. Is the allegation of negligence justified? Give reasons.

5. A young man is brought unconscious to the emergency room of a private hospital in a semi-conscious state. It is alleged that he had consumed some tablets following arguments with his female friend. An offensive odor is present at the mouth and nostrils, and the breathing is shallow and rapid. On examination signs of hypotension and pulmonary edema are present. ECG shows changes suggestive of arrhythmias.

(2 + 2 + 2 + 2 marks)

a. What can be the probable diagnosis?
b. Give reasons for your diagnosis.
c. What bedside test can be done to confirm the diagnosis?
d. What specific therapy is likely to help the patient?

6. A worker of a match factory for the last 15 years reports to the dentist with multiple sinuses and fistula formation in the jaw with foul smelling discharges.

(2 + 2 + 4 marks)

a. What is the probable diagnosis?
b. Mention the cause for the patient's condition.
c. Describe the etiopathogenesis of this condition.

7. A 30-year-old male presents to a dermatologist with diffuse alopecia of sudden onset and blurring of vision. Dermatologist notices that lateral part of eye brows and eye lashes are also missing. His wife tells the doctor about some behavioral changes she has noticed in him for the last 1–2 months. Doctor inspects the nails of the patient and comes to a diagnosis.

(2 + 2 + 2 + 2 marks)

a. What is the likely diagnosis you think the dermatologist made?
b. Give reasons for your diagnosis.
c. What changes did the doctor observe in the nails?
d. Mention other neurologic symptoms likely to be present in this case.

8. During a house fire, one of the rescue workers complained of headache, shortness of breath and dizziness. His colleagues thought he was exhausted and made him sit on one side. Very soon he had seizures and collapsed. He was rushed to emergency where he was declared brought dead. At autopsy, fine froth was present at mouth and nostrils, and postmortem staining was brick red in appearance. Autopsy surgeon subjected 5 mL of gastric contents to a quick chemical test and arrived at a provisional diagnosis.

(2 + 2 + 2 + 2 marks)

a. What is the likely diagnosis that the autopsy surgeon made?
b. Give reasons for the diagnosis.
c. What chemical test was probably performed in this case?
d. What specific therapy could have helped the patient, if he was brought to hospital earlier?

9. A young traveller presents to the emergency with history of nausea, vomiting, diarrhea, and abdominal cramps following consumption of some canned fish and sausages. There is no history of fever or loss of consciousness, but the patient complains of dryness of mouth, difficulty in swallowing and blurring of vision.

(2 + 2 + 2 + 2 marks)

a. What is the probable diagnosis?
b. What is the possible causative agent for this condition?
c. Give reasons for your diagnosis.
d. What is the specific treatment in management of this case?

10. A university student was brought to the emergency with an alleged history of consumption of some liquid that his father had brought for spraying in their fields. The patient is anxious and restless and has complaints of nausea, vomiting, diarrhea, profuse sweating and salivation. Preliminary examination shows raised BP and constricted pupils.

(2 + 2 + 2 + 2 marks)

a. What is your preliminary diagnosis?
b. Give reasons for your diagnosis.
c. What is the mechanism of action of the alleged poison?
d. Mention treatment suggested for the alleged poisoning?

11. A young man was found in a drowsy state in a bus and was brought to the emergency. The patient was muttering some indistinct and inaudible words. Flushing and hyperpyrexia was evident and the pupils were dilated. The next day he recalls of having taken some biscuits from his fellow passenger in the bus after which he did not remember anything. His valuables and luggage too were missing. Investigations confirmed that he was robbed by a gang active in the region who traps the unsuspecting victims by offering biscuits laced with a substance.

(2 + 2 + 2 + 2 marks)

a. What is your likely diagnosis?
b. Give reasons for your diagnosis.
c. Describe the mechanism of toxicity for the alleged agent.
d. How would you have managed such type of case?

12. A middle-aged female is brought to the emergency with an alleged history of snake bite on the dorsum of the hand while she was working in the farms. Her relatives have killed the snake and have brought the snake along with. The snake has a triangular head, prominent neck and a tapering tail. The dorsum of the hand shows a couple of distinct fang marks with blood oozing out.

(2 + 2 + 2 + 2 marks)

a. Identify the snake in the described case, giving suitable reasons.
b. State the type of venom injected in the case and its fatal dose.
c. How will the doctor assess the severity of snake bite in such cases?
d. Write a note on the specific therapy to be given in this case.

13. A young female presents to the emergency room with alleged history of consumption of some rodenticide. The patient is alert and conscious with complaints of recurrent convulsive episodes. The patient has never had convulsions in the past. Arching of the body is evident during the convulsive episode; otherwise, the muscles are in relaxed state.

(2 + 2 + 2 + 2 marks)

a. What is your preliminary diagnosis?
b. Give reasons for your diagnosis.
c. What is the mechanism of action of the alleged poison?
d. Mention other characteristic features likely to be present in this case.

14. On a salary day, a group of laborers go to a local liquor shop and consume a number of drinks. They were brought to emergency room in an intoxicated state with complaints of vomiting, abdominal pain, and headache. A few of them complain of blurring of vision while the others feel like "being in a snowstorm".

(2 + 2 + 2 + 2 marks)

a. What is your preliminary diagnosis?
b. Give reasons for your diagnosis.
c. What is the mechanism of action of the alleged poison?
d. Write a note on the specific therapy to be given in this case.

15. A young girl went for a bath, and she neither came out nor answered to the calls for quite some time. The door was broken and she was found unconscious in the bathroom. She was rushed to the emergency department where she was pronounced dead. At autopsy, a distinct cherry red appearance of postmortem staining and internal organs was noted. On enquiry, the parents revealed that the deceased had complained of headache and giddiness in the past especially after baths. The bathroom was poorly ventilated with a geyser installed 1 month back. Blood toxicology showed high levels of an irrespirable gas.

(2 + 2 + 4 + 4 marks)

a. What is your preliminary diagnosis?
b. Give reasons for your diagnosis.
c. What is the mechanism of action of the alleged poison?
d. Describe the clinical manifestations usually observed in such cases.

Key to Problem Based Questions

Answer 1:

a. Phenol marasmus (Chronic phenol poisoning).
b. *Reasons*: History of chronic exposure and dark urine are characteristic features.
c. Oxidation of the phenolic metabolites (hydroquinone and pyrocatechol) excreted in urine.
d. *Carbolochronosis*: Hyperpigmentation of skin and discoloration of the sclera. Hydroquinone gets deposited in the matrix of cartilage imparting a bluish gray appearance to the tissues.

Answer 2:

a. Strychnine poisoning.
b. Epileptic fits and tetanus. Differentiate with epilepsy and tetanus (*see* chapter 14 for details)
c. *Reasons*: Convulsions with arching of the body and alert and conscious state of the patient is suggestive of consumption of strychnine (a constituent of herbal medicine)
d. Supportive care (Maintain airway, breathing and circulation) and prevention and treatment of convulsions are the mainstay of treatment. Keep the patient in quiet and dark room. IV diazepam with short-acting muscle relaxants is the preferred treatment.

Answer 3:

a. Hydrogen sulfide inhalation poisoning. *Reasons*: History, offensive odor, and greenish discoloration observed at autopsy are characteristic features.
b. Respiratory arrest/Cardiac arrhythmias
c. Raised thiosulfate levels in the blood and brain and lungs are confirmatory.
d. *Antidotes*: Amyl nitrite and sodium nitrite.

Answer 4:

a. Kerosene poisoning.
b. History of exposure, symptoms of exposure and radiological observations are characteristic.
c. Airway management and oxygen therapy. Early intubation and mechanical ventilation is attempted in severe respiratory distress. Antibiotic prophylaxis may be given.
d. Yes, gastric lavage is probably responsible for worsening of patient's condition (gastric lavage is contraindicated for the risk of aspiration in poisoning with kerosene or any volatile liquids).

Answer 5:

a. Aluminium phosphide poisoning
b. *Reasons*: Offensive odor (garlicky/decaying fish odor) and ECG changes are suggestive.
c. *Silver nitrate impregnated paper test*: Filter paper impregnated with silver nitrate solution when exposed to breath/vomitus/gastric aspirate turns black as $AgNO_3$ is reduced to Ag. On adding a drop of ammonium molybdate solution, black filter paper turns blue.
d. Intravenous infusion of magnesium sulfate is suggested as specific therapy (Magnesium sulfate to correct hypomagnesemia and for effective management of arrhythmias).

Answer 6:

a. Phossy jaw (Chronic phosphorus poisoning)
b. Chronic exposure to white/yellow phosphorus fumes
c. Etiopathogenesis: (*see* Flowchart 1 in Chapter 6 for details).

Answer 7:

a. Thallium poisoning.

b. *Reason*: Diffuse alopecia of sudden onset and loss of eye brows (typically the lateral part), and eye lashes along with diplopia (blurring of vision) are suggestive.
c. Mee's lines in the nail plate (transverse white lines on the nails) were observed by the doctor.
d. Ascending peripheral neuropathies are reported. Pain and paresthesias of the extremities is common. Distal motor weakness occurs predominantly of the lower limbs.

Answer 8:

a. Cyanide poisoning.
b. *Reasons*: History of exposure, symptoms, and characteristic color of postmortem lividity.
c. *Lee Jones test*: 5 mL of gastric aspirate + few Fe_2SO_4 crystals + 5 drops of NaOH solution; Boil, then cool and add few drops of 10% HCl; Greenish blue precipitate is suggestive of the presence of cyanide.
d. Antidotal therapy (Eli-Lilly cyanide antidote kit/3-step cyanide antidote kit) is the specific treatment (*see* chapter 16 on cyanide poisoning for details).

Answer 9:

a. Foodborne botulism
b. *Clostridium botulinum* (a gram positive, spore forming anaerobic bacilli)
c. *Reasons*: History and characteristic symptoms such as blurring of vision (diplopia), dryness of mouth, dysphagia (difficulty in swallowing), etc.
d. Trivalent antitoxin (A, B, and E) is the specific treatment, and should be administered at the earliest.

Answer 10:

a. Organophosphate compound (OPC) poisoning
b. *Reasons*: History and symptoms (Muscarinic, nicotinic and early CNS effects) are suggestive.
c. *Mechanism of action:* Organophosphate compounds act by inhibition of cholinesterase (ChE) enzyme (*see* chapter 18 for details)
d. Atropine together with oximes is the most effective therapy in organophosphate poisoning (*see* chapter 18 for details).

Answer 11:

a. Datura poisoning.
b. *Reasons*: History of the case; symptoms such as dilated pupils, flushing, hyperpyrexia, drowsiness and muttering delirium are suggestive of datura poisoning.
c. *Mechanism of action:* The alkaloids of datura competitively block the neurotransmitter acetylcholine at muscarinic receptor, centrally and peripherally, and also at end organ sites of parasympathetic nervous system. The stage of overstimulation of the nervous system is followed by the stage of depression. Scopolamine crosses blood brain barrier and is responsible for the CNS effects like delirium, drowsiness, agitation and dementia.
d. Physostigmine is the specific treatment. Besides, symptomatic and supportive treatment in form of artificial respiration, oxygen inhalation (for patients with respiratory depression), sponging (for dry skin and to bring down the high temperature), and benzodiazepines (to control agitation) would be useful in treating such a case.

Answer 12:

a. Viper. *Reasons*: Description of the snake and the local examination.
b. *Vasculotoxin; fatal dose*: 20 mg (Russell's viper) or 8 mg (Saw-scaled viper).

c. Severity assessment (*see* chapter 9 for details).
d. Antivenom therapy is the specific antidote/treatment of choice (*see* chapter 9 for details).

Answer 13:

a. Strychnine poisoning.
b. *Reasons*: Convulsions with arching of the body and alert and conscious state of the patient is suggestive of consumption of strychnine (a constituent of rodenticides)
c. *Mechanism of action:* Strychnine acts as an antagonist of inhibitory neurotransmitter glycine. It blocks the receptors preventing the postsynaptic uptake of glycine by brain stem and spinal cord. The widespread inhibition results in increased reflex excitability.
d. Opisthotonus/Emprosthotonus/Pleurosthotonus, Hippus, Risus Sardonicus/Satan's face/Sardonic grin (Devilish grin), etc.

Answer 14:

a. Methanol poisoning.
b. *Reasons*: History and symptoms (blurring of vision especially that of "like being in a snowstorm") are characteristic of methanol intoxication.
c. *Mechanism of action:* Methanol is oxidized to formaldehyde first and then to formic acid by enzyme dehydrogenases. The metabolites of methanol: formaldehyde and formic acid (predominantly) are responsible for its toxic effects. Methanol → Formaldehyde → Formic acid (*see* chapter 11 for details).
d. Specific therapy includes ethanol and fomepizole (*see* chapter 11 for details).

Answer 15:

a. Carbon monoxide poisoning.
b. *Reasons*: History (gas geyser in a poorly ventilated bathroom) and symptoms (characteristic appearance of lividity and organs at autopsy) are characteristics of carbon monoxide poisoning.
c. *Mechanism of action*: CO is rapidly absorbed by the lungs. The affinity of CO to hemoglobin (Hb) is 200–250 times greater than oxygen. Hence, it readily binds to Hb and forms carboxyhemoglobin (COHb) resulting in anemic anoxia/hypoxia. Likewise, CO also binds to myoglobin (60 times greater affinity than O_2). With increasing levels of COHb, there is a leftward shift of the oxyhemoglobin dissociation curve. CO also affects the intracellular respiration by blocking cytochrome oxidase and cytochrome P450, etc.
d. *Clinical manifestations*: Vary with the COHb concentrations (Table 1).

Table 1: Clinical manifestations of carbon monoxide poisoning

COHb%	Clinical manifestations
0–10	Asymptomatic
10–20	Mild headache, breathlessness on exertion
20–30	Throbbing headache, irritability, fatigue, emotional instability
30–40	Severe headache, nausea, vomiting, dizziness, dimness of vision, tinnitus, confusion, and cherry red discoloration of skin
40–50	Increasing confusion, ataxia, rapid respiration, hallucinations, and muscle incoordination Symptoms resemble alcohol intoxication
50–60	Pink or red discoloration of skin, rapid respiration, tachycardia, convulsions, and coma
>60	Skin blisters (cutaneous bullae), deep coma, arrhythmias, and death

Quick Facts: Time to Revise Important Points

CHAPTER 24

"*Paracelsus*" is considered as the father of toxicology.

"*Mathieu Orfila*" is considered as the father of modern toxicology.

Mechanism of Action of Some Common Poisons

- *Methanol/Ethanol*: Oxidation to aldehyde and acid by enzyme dehydrogenases.
- *Datura*: Blocking of the neurotransmitter acetylcholine.
- *Strychnine*: Antagonism of inhibitory neurotransmitter glycine (action at anterior horn cells)
- *Aconite*: Persistent activation of the sodium channels
- *Carbon monoxide*: Greater affinity to Hb forming COHb, causing *anemic anoxia/hypoxia*. It blocks cytochrome oxidase and cytochrome P450 affecting the intracellular respiration.
- *Cyanide*: Inhibition of enzyme systems of cellular respiration (cytochrome oxidase, carbonic anhydrase, etc.). Large doses cause *histotoxic anoxia* (i.e. prevents cells from using oxygen).
- *Organophosphorous compounds*: Cholinesterase enzyme inhibition, limiting the degradation of ACh causing excess accumulation of Ach and overstimulation of ACh receptors at synapses.
- *Aluminum/Zinc phosphide*: Release of highly toxic phosphine gas (PH_3) on exposure to moisture or by the action of hydrochloric acid in the stomach. It blocks the enzyme cytochrome C oxidase, thus, inhibiting the mitochondrial oxidative phosphorylation. Mitochondrial cytochrome C oxidase inhibition causes cellular hypoxia and results in widespread organ damage (Cytotoxic phosphine gas).
- *Botulinum toxin:* Is a neurotoxin that acts by presynaptic binding to cholinergic nerve fibers. The toxin inhibits the release of acetylcholine from nerve terminals causing flaccid paralysis.
- *Lead*: Lead inhibits enzymes aminolevulinic acid (ALA) dehydratase, coproporphyrinogen oxidase, and ferrochalatase resulting in inhibition of heme synthesis.

Table 1: Specific toxicity of certain poisons

Kerosene	Pulmonary toxicity (Chemical/Aspiration pneumonitis)
Methanol	Ocular toxicity (Retinal damage and blindness), renal toxicity
Paraquat	Pulmonary toxicity (Progressive pulmonary fibrosis; Paraquat lung)
Carbolic and Oxalic Acid	Renal toxicity

Table 2: Common poisons and their antidotes

Poisoning	*Antidotes*
Benzodiazepines	Flumazenil
Botulism	Trivalent antitoxin (A, B, and E)
Carbon monoxide	Oxygen
Carbamates	Atropine
Cyanides	Cyanide antidote kit (amyl nitrite, sodium nitrite, thiosulphate)
Datura	Physostigmine
Ethylene glycol	Ethanol, fomepizole
Heavy metals (in general)	Chelating agents
• Arsenic, mercury	• BAL, EDTA
• Copper	• Penicillamine
• Iron	• Deferoxamine
• Lead	• EDTA, BAL
Methanol	Ethanol, Fomepizole
Morphine/Opium	Naloxone
Organophosphates	Atropine, oximes
Paracetamol	N-acetyl cysteine
Phosphorus	Copper sulfate
Snake bite	Polyvalent ASV
Thallium	Prussian blue
Mushroom poisoning	Atropine
Nicotine addiction	Bupropion, clonidine, nicotine gum
Opioid addiction	Methadone
Chronic alcoholism	Disulfiram (Antabuse)

Table 3: Potentially toxic antidotes

Antidote (Potentially toxic)	*Used in poisoning of*
Amyl nitrite	Cyanide
Atropine	Organophosphates
Barbiturates	Strychnine
Chelating agents	Heavy metals
Copper sulfate	Phosphorous
Ethanol	Methanol and ethylene glycol
Potassium permanganate	Phosphorus, opium, strychnine

Table 4: Characteristic symptoms and associated poisoning

Clinical condition/disease	*Poisoning*
Dilated pupils	Alcohol, datura, cannabis, cocaine, LSD
Constricted pupils	Opium, phenol, alcohol coma, carbamate, OPC
Hippus	Aconite, strychnine
Macewen's sign	Ethyl alcohol
Mee's line on nails	Chronic arsenic, thallium
Basophilic stippling	Chronic lead
Burtonian/Burton's line (Blue line on gums)	Chronic lead (Also in mercury, copper, bismuth)
Flea bitten appearance of the GI mucosa	Arsenic (Red velvety appearance/congestion)
Horizontal gaze nystagmus	Ethyl alcohol, MDMA, barbiturates
Horizontal and vertical gaze nystagmus	Phencyclidine (PCP)
Neurolathyrism	*Lathyrus sativus*
Epidemic dropsy	*Argemone mexicana*
Opisthotonus, pleurosthotonus, emprosthotonus	Strychnine
Phossy jaw	Phosphorus
Oxaluria	Oxalic acid, ethylene glycol
Carboluria	Phenol/Carbolic acid
Oochronosis	Phenol/Carbolic acid
Magnan's phenomenon/Formication	Cocaine
Amotivational syndrome	Chronic cannabis
Run Amok/Running Amok	Chronic cannabis
Hashish/Charas/Hemp insanity	Chronic cannabis
Flash back phenomenon	LSD
Mercuria lentis	Mercury (anterior lens capsule pigmentation)
Minamata disease	Organic mercury
Peripheral neuropathy and alopecia	Thallium
Priapism (painful prolonged penile erection)	Cantharides, scorpion sting envenomation
Black foot disease	Arsenic
Bhopal gas tragedy/Bhopal disaster	Methyl icocyanate (MIC) gas
Metal fume fever/brass chills	Metal (Zn, Cu, Hg, Pb, Sb, etc.) oxide inhalation
Strawberry tongue	Acute mercury

Table 5: Typical odor characteristic of poisoning

Odor	*Poison*
Bitter almond	Cyanide, hydrogen cyanide, nitrobenzene
Burnt rope	Cannabis
Garlic/garlicky	Phosphorus, organophosphates, thalllium, arsenic
Fishy	Zinc and aluminium phosphide
Rotten egg	Hydrogen sulfide
Fruity	Alcohol, solvents
Sweet	Chloroform (halogenated hydrocarbons)
Kerosene like	Kerosene, organophosphates/carbamates (solvents)
Phenolic	Carbolic acid, lysol, etc.

Table 6: Postmortem lividity characteristic of poisoning

Postmortem lividity	Poisoning
Gray-brown/Chocolate	Aniline, nitrites, nitrates
Cherry red/Light red	Carbon monoxide
Brick pink/Brick red	Cyanide
Dark/Black	Opium
Brown/Yellow-brown	Phosphorus
Bluish green	Hydrogen sulfide

Table 7: Poisoning where clinical manifestations resemble natural diseases

Acute mercury poisoning	Diphtheric colitis involving the ascending and transverse colon
Acute arsenic poisoning	Cholera
Acute arsenic poisoning	Acute yellow fatty liver
Acute phosphorus poisoning	Acute yellow atrophy of liver
Mild CO poisoning	Flu-like syndromes
Thallium poisoning	Guillain-Barré syndrome
Cardiotoxic agents	Arrhythmias/Heart disease
Strychnine poisoning	Tetanus, Epilepsy

Table 8: Syndromes in toxicology

Smoky/Smoking stools syndrome	Acute phosphorus poisoning
Fanconi's syndrome	Acute lead (Pb) poisoning
Body packer syndrome	Cocaine/heroin drug carriers
Mallory-Weiss syndrome	Alcoholism
Fetal alcohol syndrome	Alcohol abuse during pregnancy
Marchiafava-Bignami syndrome	Alcohol abuse
Wernicke-Korsakoff syndrome	Alcohol abuse
Aldehyde syndrome	Disulfiram treatment
Auto brewery syndrome	Endogenous production of alcohol
Amotivational syndrome	Chronic cannabis poisoning
Intermediate syndrome	Type II paralysis in organophosphate poisoning
Phalloides syndrome	Mushroom *(Amanita phalloides)* poisoning
Holiday heart syndrome	Atrial fibrillation (AF) after an alcohol binge

Table 9: Commonly used names/ slang for certain compounds and their mixture

Speed balls	Mixture of cocaine and heroin
Micky finn	Solution of chloral hydrate and alcohol
Knock out drops	Solution of chloral hydrate and alcohol
Angel dust	Phencyclidine (PCP)
Liquid gold	Urine of amphetamine addicts
Brown sugar, black tar	Popular forms of heroin among addicts
Ecstasy	MDMA (Methylene-dioxy-methamphetamine)
Plant penicillin	Endrin
Ghazipur opium	Standardized opium (10% morphine) produced at Ghazipur
Hyderabadi goli	Capsicum
Mitha bish	Aconite

Table 10: Potentially toxic plants and their active ingredients

Plant irritants	*Active ingredients (alkaloids/active principles)*
Abrus precatorius	Abrin, abrine, abraline, abric acid, abrussic acid
Ricinus communis	Ricin, ricinine
Croton tiglium	Crotin, crotonoside, crotonoleic acid
Semecarpus anacardium	Bhilawanol, semecarpol
Calotropis gigantea	Calactin, calotoxin, calotropin, uscharin, gigantin
Calotropis procera	Calactin, calotoxin, calotropin, uscharin
Plumbago rosea	Plumbagin
Capsicum annum	Capsaicin, capsicin
Aconitum ferox/napellus	Aconitine (Locally actively irritant; otherwise broadly has cardiotoxic properties)
Cardiotoxic plants	
Nicotiana tabacum	Nicotine, anabasine, nicotianine, lobeline
Nerium oleander/odorum	Nerine, nerioside, folinerin, rosagenin, oleandrin
Cerbera thevetia	Cerberin, thevetin, thevetoxin, nerifolin
Cerbera odallum	Cerberin, odollin, odolotoxin, thevetin
Aconitum ferox/napellus	Aconitine, mesaconitine, hypaconitine bikhaconitine, indaconitine, picraconitine
Digitalis purpurea	Digitoxin, digitalin, digoxin
Cinchona officinalis	Quinine, quinidine, cinchonine
Neurotoxic agents	
Datura alba	Hyoscine (scopolamine), hyoscyamine, traces of atropine
Cannabis indica	Cannabinoids: cannabinol, cannabidiol The active form is Δ-9 tetrahydrocannabinol (THC)
Papaver somniferum (Opium)	• *Phenanthrene alkaloids:* Morphine, codeine, thebaine • *Benzyl-isoquinoline alkaloids:* Papaverine, noscapine
Adulterants	
Argemone mexicana	Sanguinarine and dihydrosanguinarine in oil
Lathyrus sativus	BOAA (β-N-oxalyl amino alanine) in seeds

Psychiatric Manifestations Associated with Poisonings

- *Delirium tremens*: An acute episode of delirium in alcohol withdrawal
- *Muttering delirium*: Datura poisoning (Delirious victim mutters indistinct/inaudible words)
- *Carphologia and pill rolling*: Datura poisoning (Purpose less movements of delirious victim like pulling imaginary threads (*carphologia*), threading imaginary needle (*pill rolling*).
- *Hallucinations*:
  - *Visual/Auditory hallucinations*: In poisoning with mercury, morphine, datura, cannabis, cocaine, carbon monoxide (COHb 40–50%) and alcohol withdrawal syndrome
  - *Lilliputian hallucinations/Microptic hallucinations*: In acute cocaine poisoning
  - *Tactile hallucinations/Cocaine bug/Coke bug/Magnan's symptoms/Magnan's phenomenon/Magnan-Saury's sign/Formication/Formicative hallucination/Insect hallucination*: In cocaine intoxication.
  - *Visual hallucinations and illusion*: In LSD and phencyclidine (PCP).

Common Tests in Toxicology

- *Lee Jones test is a rapid bedside test*: 5 mL of gastric aspirate + few Fe_2SO_4 crystals + 5 drops of NaOH solution; boil, then cool and add few drops of 10% HCl **Greenish blue** precipitate is suggestive of cyanide poisoning.
- *Silver nitrate impregnated paper test*: Filter paper impregnated with silver nitrate solution when exposed to breath/vomitus/gastric aspirate turns **black** as $AgNO_3$ is reduced to Ag. On adding a drop of ammonium molybdate solution, black filter paper turns **blue**, suggestive of aluminium phosphide poisoning.
- *Marquis test*: A mixture of 3 mL concentrated H_2SO_4 and three drops of formalin is added to the sample to be analyzed. Color changes to **purple** followed by **black**, if sample is positive for morphine.
- *Reinsch's test, Marsh's test*: For chronic arsenic exposure.
- *Breath test/Breath analyzer test*: For estimating the blood alcohol content (BAC). Potassium dichromate crystals/solutions were used in the breath analyzers. Reaction of alcohol with potassium dichromate (*red orange*) brings about color changes due to formation of chromium sulfate (**green**).

Full/Expanded Forms

- BAL (British Anti-Lewisite)
- EDTA (Ethylene diamine tetraacetic acid)
- DMPS (Dimercapto-propane sulfonate)
- DMSA (Dimercapto-succinic acid)
- DDT (Dichloro-diphenyl-trichloroethane)
- MDMA (Methylene-dioxy-methamphetamine)
- LSD (Lysergic acid diethylamide)

Important Legal Provisions in Toxicology

CrPC (The Code of Criminal Procedure, 1973):

- *Section 39 Cr PC*: Doctor is legally bound to report homicidal poisoning and offences relating to adulteration of food and drugs, etc. to police/magistrate
- *Section 53 Cr PC*: *"Examination of accused by medical practitioner at the request of police officer"* (consent is not mandatory for examination of an arrested person for drunkenness)
- *Section 175 Cr PC*: Investigating officer has the power to summon the doctor and seek relevant information about any MLC, including the poisoning cases.

IPC (The Indian Penal Code, 1860):

- *Section 85 IPC*: *"Act of a person incapable of judgment by reason of intoxication caused against his will"*
- *Section 86 IPC*: *"Offence requiring a particular intent or knowledge committed by one who is intoxicated"*
- *Section 176 IPC*: *"Omission to give notice or information to public servant by person legally bound to give it"* (Failure on part of doctor to inform the police is punishable).
- *Section 201 IPC*: *"Causing disappearance of evidence of offence, or giving false information to screen offender"* (Failure on part of doctor to preserve samples is punishable).
- *Section 202 IPC*: *"Intentional omission to give information of offence by person bound to inform."* (Intentional omission to give information by the doctor is punishable).
- *Section 326A and 326B (Inserted to Section 326 IPC)*: For stricter punishments for offences related to vitriolage, etc. Corrosives are included as dangerous weapon/means.

MVA (The Motor Vehicles Act, 1988):

- *Section 185 MVA*: Driving by a drunken person or by a person under the influence of drugs is a punishable offence in India.
- *Section 202-205 MVA*: Deals with medical examination, breath test and laboratory tests in cases of drunken driving.

Table 11: Fatal dose (approximate) in some common poisonings

Poisoning	Fatal dose
Mineral acids	10–20 mL
Arsenic trioxide	0.1–0.2 g
Lead/mercury/copper salts	20–40 g
Plant irritants	
• Abrus	1–2 crushed seeds (100–120 mg abrin)
• Croton	4–5 crushed seeds (4–5 ml croton oil)
• Ricinus	8–10 crushed seeds (6 mg ricin)
Snake bite (dried venom)	
• Krait	6 mg
• King cobra	12 mg
• Cobra	15 mg
• Saw-scaled viper	8 mg
• Russell's viper	20 mg
Opium	2 g (Morphine: 0.2 g orally/0.1 g parenterally)
Alcohol	
• Ethanol	BAC > 500 mg%, 150–250 ml of absolute alcohol taken in 1 hour
• Methanol	BAC 200 mg%, 60–250 mL
Datura	50–100 seeds
Cannabis products	
• Bhang	10 g/kg body weight
• Ganja	8 g/kg body weight
• Charas/Hashish	2 g/kg body weight
Strychnous nux vomica	1–3 crushed seeds (20–50 mg of strychnine)
Aconitine	3–6 g
Carbon monoxide	COHb > 60%
Cyanide	
• Pure HCN	50–100 mg
• NaCN/ KCN	200–300 mg
Nicotine	50–100 mg
Crude tobacco	15–30 g
Aluminum phosphide	1–3 tablets

Table 12: Revise the mnemonics

Mnemonic	Reference	Page for details
CINCAMS	Classification of poisons	4
5Is or IIIII	Routes of exposure of poisoning	6
COAL	Abortifacients	5
ABCD	Stupefying agents	5
ABCD	Dilated pupils	9
OPC-OPC	Constricted pupils	9
ABCDE-DAS	Principles of management of poisoning (Manage Airway, Breathing, Circulation, Depression of CNS, Exposure reduction-Decontamination, Antidotes, Symptomatic and Supportive)	9
NDT or Do Not Trouble	Coma cocktail	10
LAST Barb 'or' BLAST	Poisons treated by hemodialysis	11
C except C	Absolute contraindication of gastric lavage	13
CHECK CC	Relative contraindication of gastric lavage	13
ATM 211	Constituents of universal antidote in ratio	16
DIP C DAD	Legal duties of a doctor in a case of poisoning	20–21
SLUDGE	Clinical features of mineral acid poisoning	23
CARBOL	Clinical features of carbolic acid poisoning	27
POTA	Poisons that give garlicky odor	9
P4	Characteristics of phosphorus poisoning	33
ARSENIC	Clinical manifestations of chronic arsenic poisoning	37
ABCDEF or Pb Lead	Clinical manifestations of chronic lead poisoning	38
Hg-MERCURI	Clinical manifestations of chronic mercury poisoning	41
GET	Triad of chronic mercury poisoning	40
9Ps	Manifestation of Pink's disease/Acrodynia	41
3As	Triad of thallium poisoning	42
ARC or CAR	Name of some toxalbumins	44
SCARPEAN	Clinical manifestations in scorpion bite	55
ABCDEFGH M4	Manifestations of chronic alcoholism	66–67
WITHDRAW	Alcohol withdrawal symptoms	68
12 Ds	Manifestations of datura poisoning	77
A to H, O to T	Manifestations of strychnine poisoning	87
DUMBBELLS	Muscarinic effects in organophosphate poisoning	103
MATCH	Nicotinic effects in organophosphate poisoning	103
RASH CAT	Early CNS effects in organophosphate poisoning	103
ARC CC	Late CNS effects in organophosphate poisoning	103
8Ds and 4Bs	Manifestations of botulism toxicity	117
PIC	Objectives of Poison Information Center	125

CHAPTER 25

Examination Time: Very Commonly Asked Questions

Descriptive/Long Questions

Mechanism of action, clinical manifestations, management, autopsy findings and medicolegal significance of:

	Page no. for details
• Aluminium phosphide poisoning	107
• Carbon monoxide poisoning	92
• Chronic arsenic poisoning	37
• Chronic lead poisoning	38
• Cyanide poisoning	94
• Opium poisoning	57
• Organophosphate poisoning	101
• Methyl alcohol poisoning	73
• *Strychnos nux vomica* poisoning	86

Mention the Differences Between

	Page no. for details
• Acute arsenic poisoning versus cholera	34
• Body packers versus body stuffers	114
• Corrosive acids versus corrosive alkalis	22
• Cobra versus viper	50
• Corrosive mineral acids (H_2SO_4 versus HNO_3 versus HCl)	23
• Datura seeds versus chilli seeds	78
• Drug addiction versus drug habituation	112
• Strychnine poisoning versus tetanus	89
• True bruise versus artificial bruise	46
• Venomous versus nonvenomous snakes	49
• White/Yellow versus red phosphorus	31

Write Short Notes

Topic	Page no.	Topic	Page no.
• Antidotes	15	• Food poisoning	116
• Body packer syndrome	114	• Factors modifying action of poison	7
• Botulism	116	• Hydrargyrism	40
• Carbamate poisoning	106	• Kerosene poisoning	123
• Carbolism	27	• Lathyrism	119
• Chelating agents	16	• Legal duties of medical practitioner	20
• Date rape drugs	115	• Methanol intoxication	73
• Datura poisoning	76	• Oxalic acid poisoning	28
• Delirium tremens	68	• Plumbism	38
• Designer drugs	83	• Poison information center	125
• Drug dependence	111	• Vitriolage	25
• Drunkenness	69	• Wernicke-Korsakoff syndrome	67
• Ethylene glycol poisoning	75	• War gases	100

Very Commonly Asked in Viva-voce

(Refer to respective chapters to find the details of the topics mentioned in Table 1. May use subject index to ease your search)

Table 1: Commonly asked questions in viva-voce

Level: Mild	*Level: Moderate to severe*
What is toxicology	Plumbism
Define poison and routes of poisoning	Carboluria and oxaluria
Antidote and its types	Hydrargyrism
Classify poisons	Drug addiction vs drug habituation
Vitriolage	Basophilic stippling
Contraindications of gastric lavage	Permissible BAC in India
Chelating agents (Definition and examples)	Levels of COHb and symptoms caused
Toxalbumins (Definition and examples)	Oochronosis
Antidotes for different poisons	Coma Cocktail
Pupillary changes (Dilatation/constriction)	Atropinization
MacEwen's sign	Management of cyanide poisoning
Hippus	Minamata disease
Types of venom of snakes	Lathyrism
Sui: Preparation and medicolegal importance	Body packers versus stuffers
Universal antidote	Tests for drunkenness
Active principles of plant irritants	Wernicke-Korsakoff syndrome
Specific features: Chronic arsenic poisoning	Hashish insanity
Specific features: Chronic mercury poisoning	Cholinesterases
Specific features: Chronic lead poisoning	Fatal doses of poisons
Manifestations of datura poisoning	Widmark formula

Contd...

Contd...

Level: Mild	*Level: Moderate to severe*
Legal duties of doctor in case of poisoning	Date rape drugs
Formication/Magnan's symptoms	Designer drugs
Manifestations of Strychnine poisoning	Warfare agents/War gases
Typical odor in different poisoning	Different syndromes (see quick facts)
PM staining in different poisonings	Specific features: Thallium poisoning
Mechanism of action of different poisons	Intermediate syndrome
Differences (Poisonings vs natural diseases)	Ghost wells
Mee's lines/Burton's lines/Blue lines	Metal fume fever
Specific toxicity of different poisons	Mania a potu
Phossy jaw cause and etiopathogenesis	Ghazipur opium'
Run amok	Hyderabadi goli
Management of snake bite envenomation	Hunan hand
Acrodynia/Pink disease	Breath analyzer test

Appliances and Spotters in Practical Examinations

CHAPTER 26

This chapter is meant for identification and quick revision of "Spotters" before examinations.

Common Appliances Used in Management of Poisoning

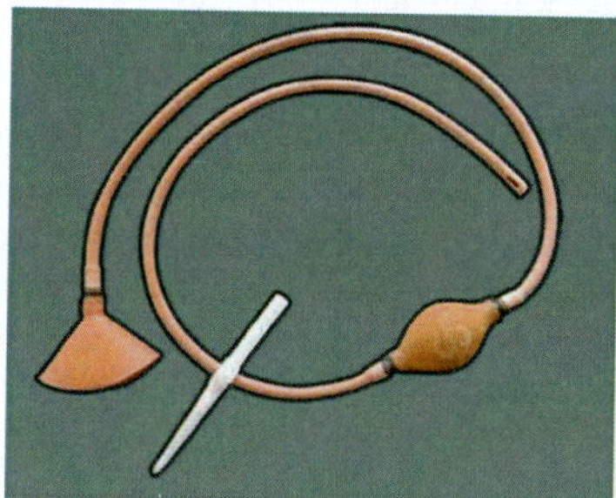

Gastric lavage tube

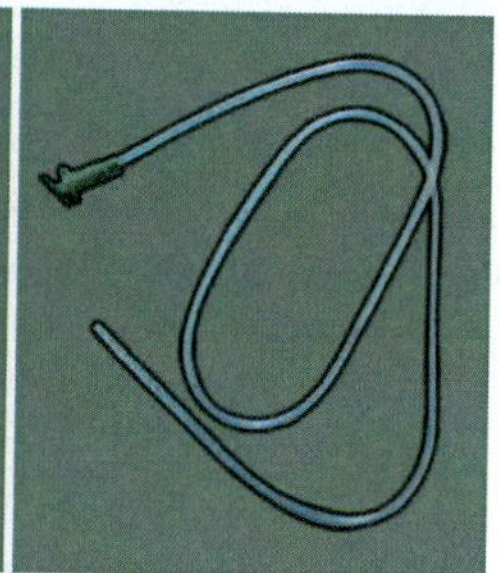

Ryle's tube

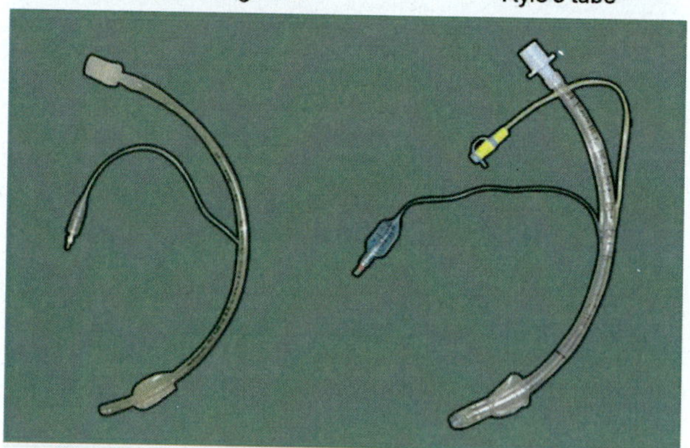

Endotracheal tubes

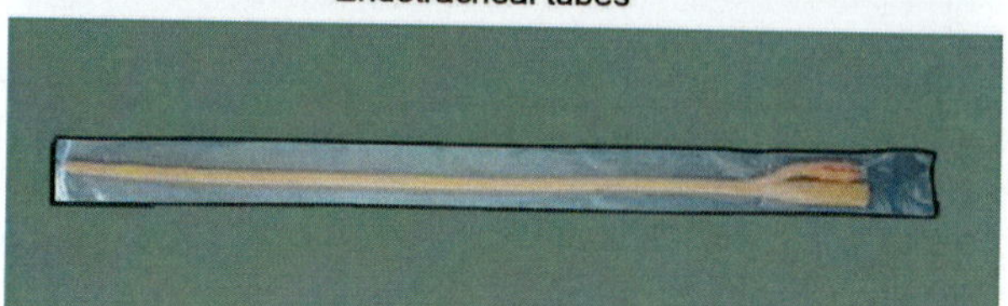

Foley catheter

Common Poisonous Plants and their Parts

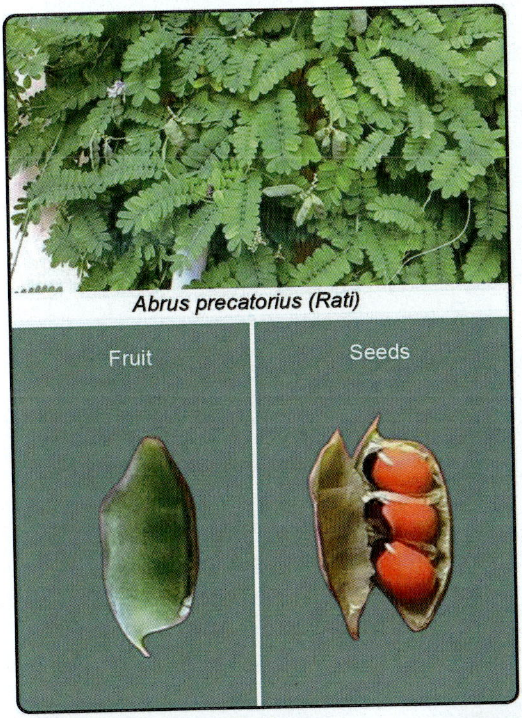
Fruit
Seeds

Abrus precatorius (Rati)

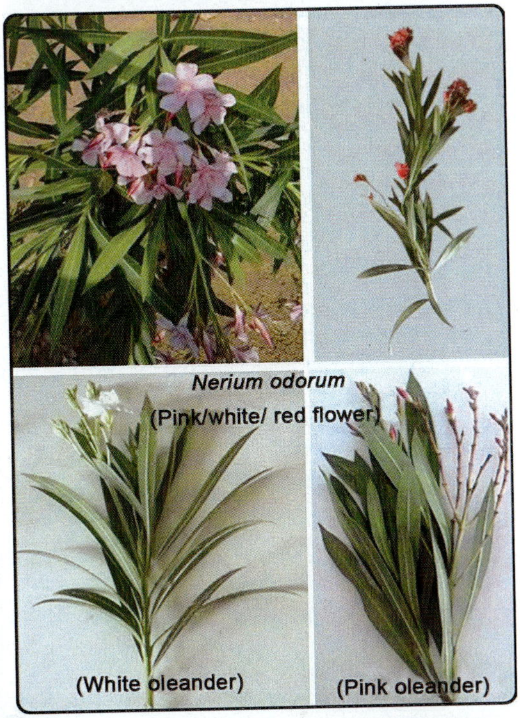
(White oleander)
(Pink oleander)

Nerium odorum
(Pink/white/ red flower)

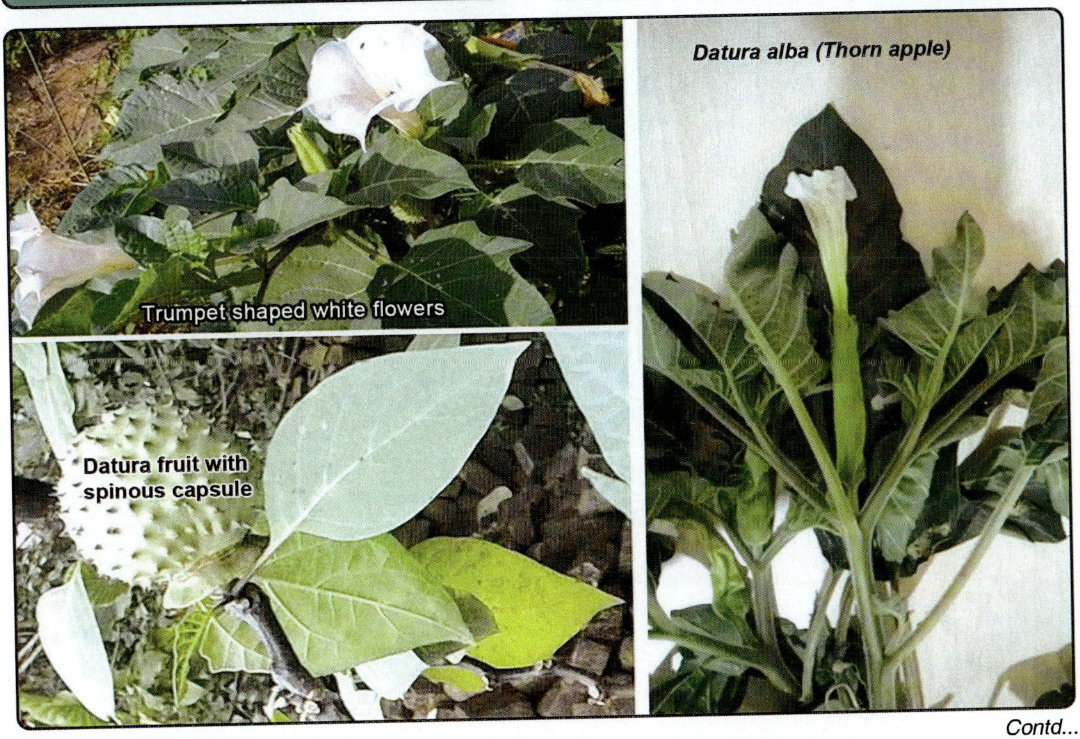
Trumpet shaped white flowers
Datura fruit with spinous capsule

Datura alba (Thorn apple)

Contd...

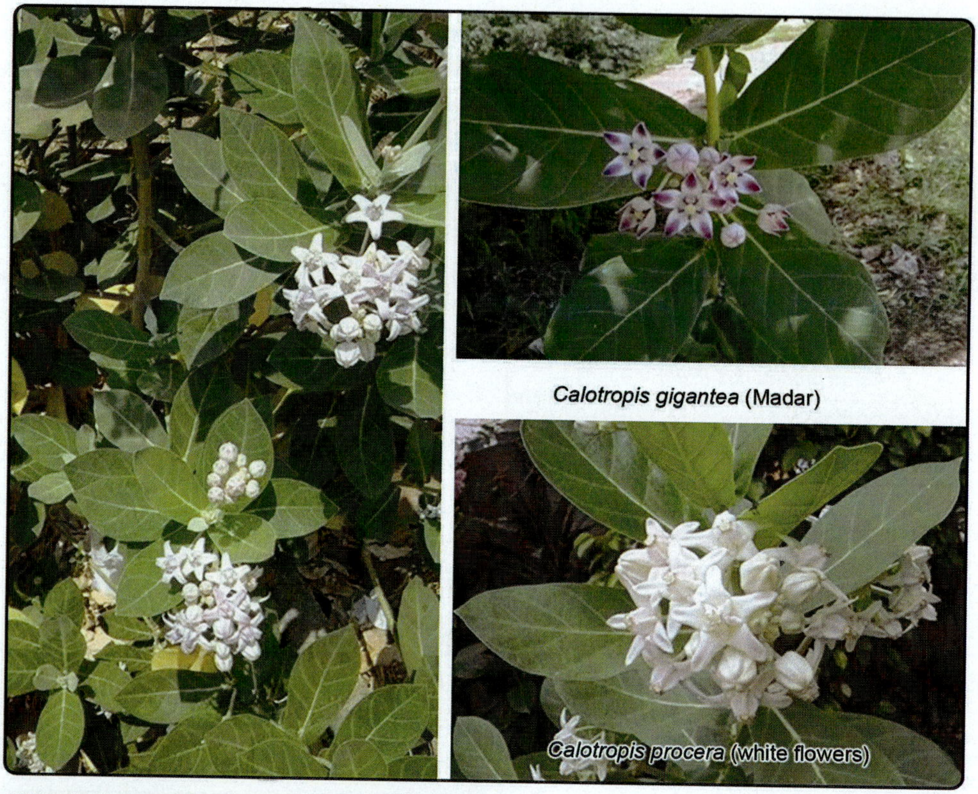
Calotropis gigantea (Madar)
Calotropis procera (white flowers)

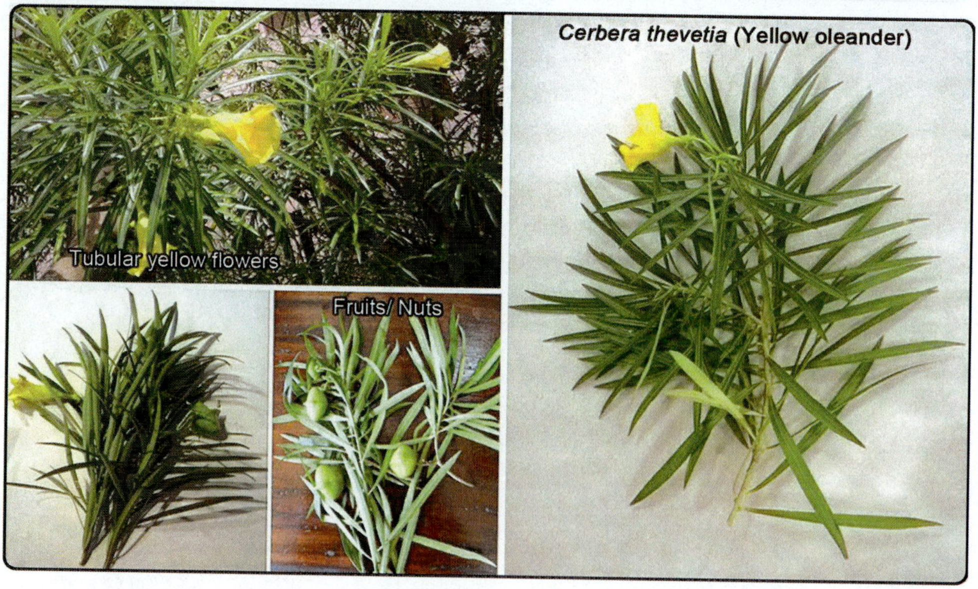
Cerbera thevetia (Yellow oleander)
Tubular yellow flowers
Fruits/ Nuts

Contd...

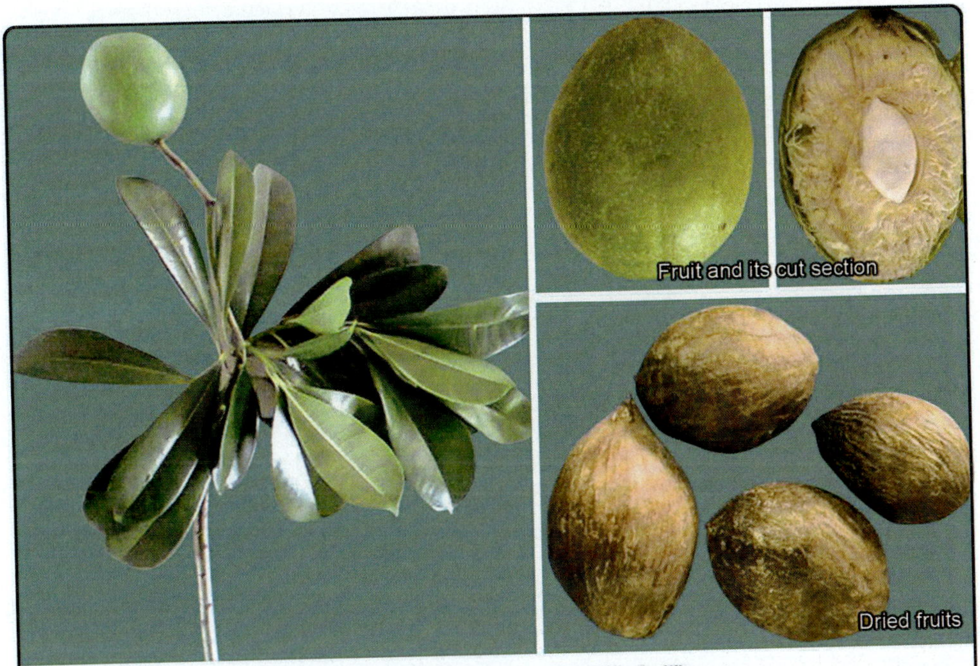

Cerbera odollam (The 'Suicide tree' / 'Suicide fruit')

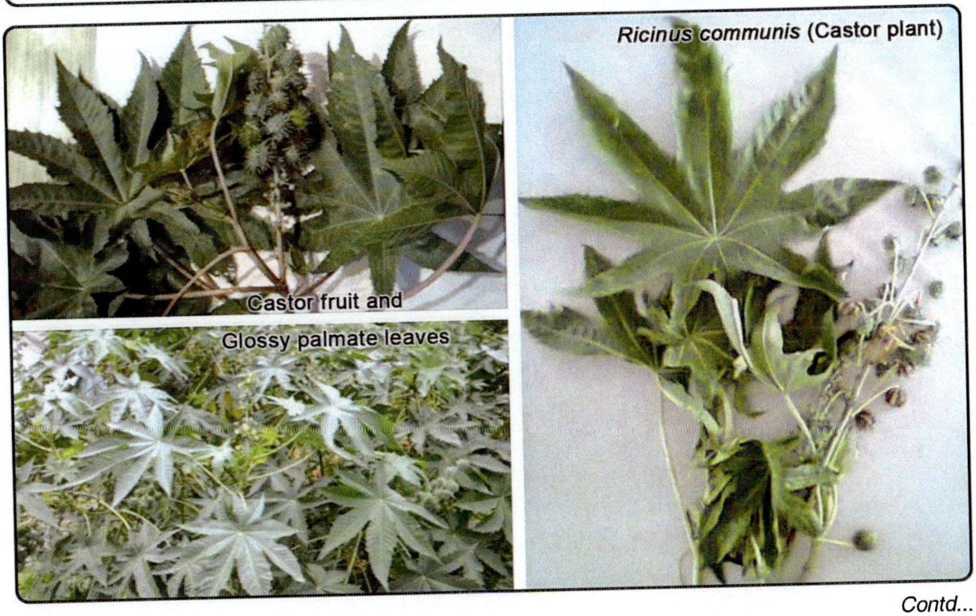

Ricinus communis (Castor plant)

Contd...

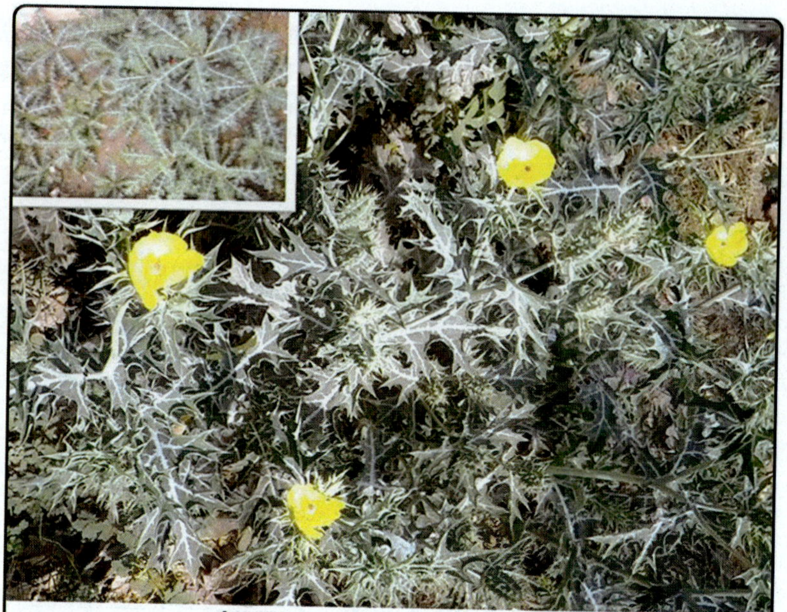

Argemone mexicana (Satyanashi)

Contd...

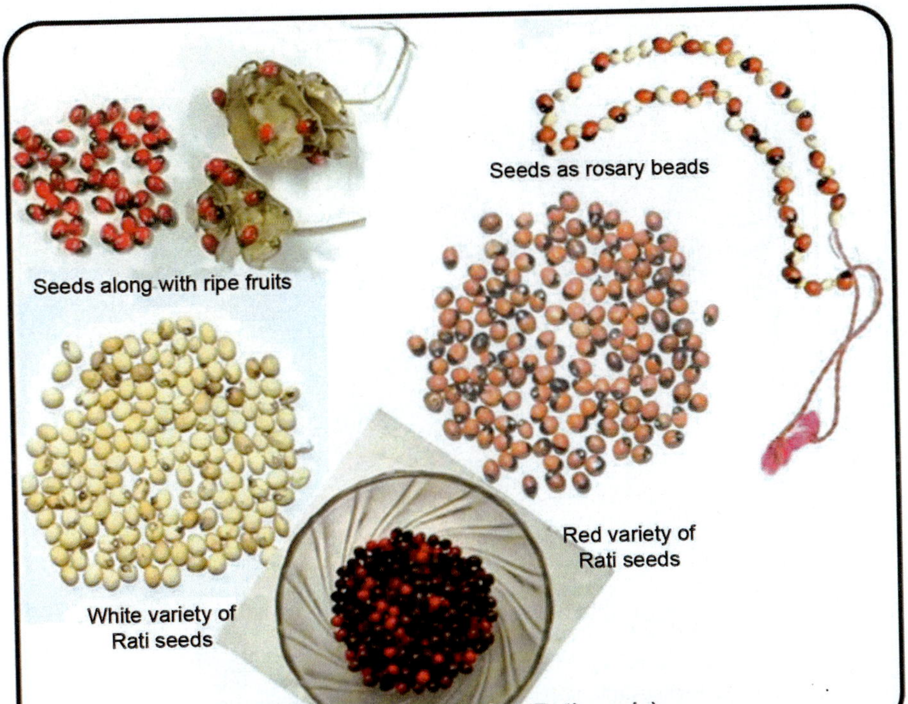

Seeds of *Abrus precatorius* (Rati seeds)

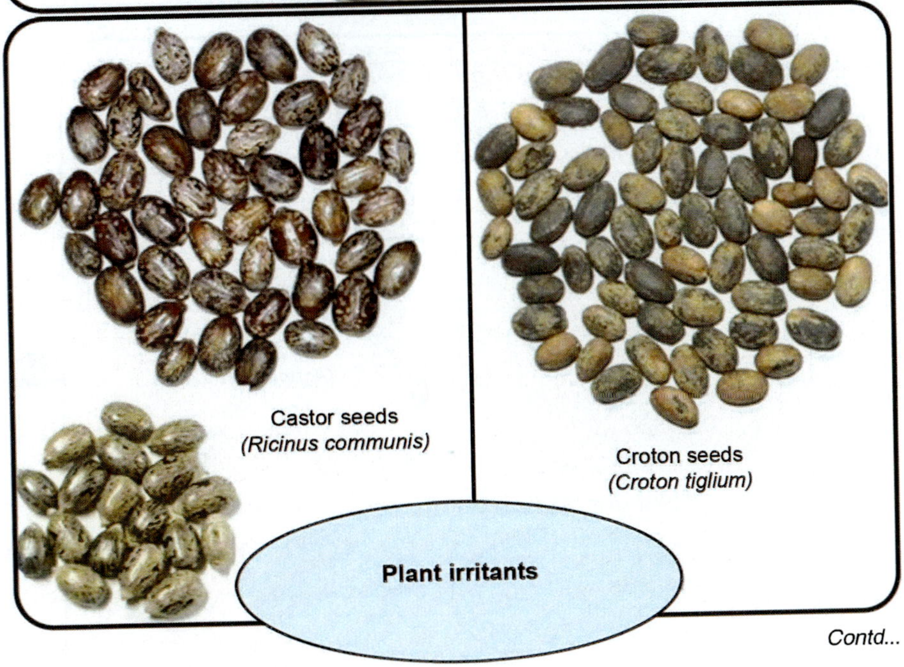

Plant irritants

Contd...

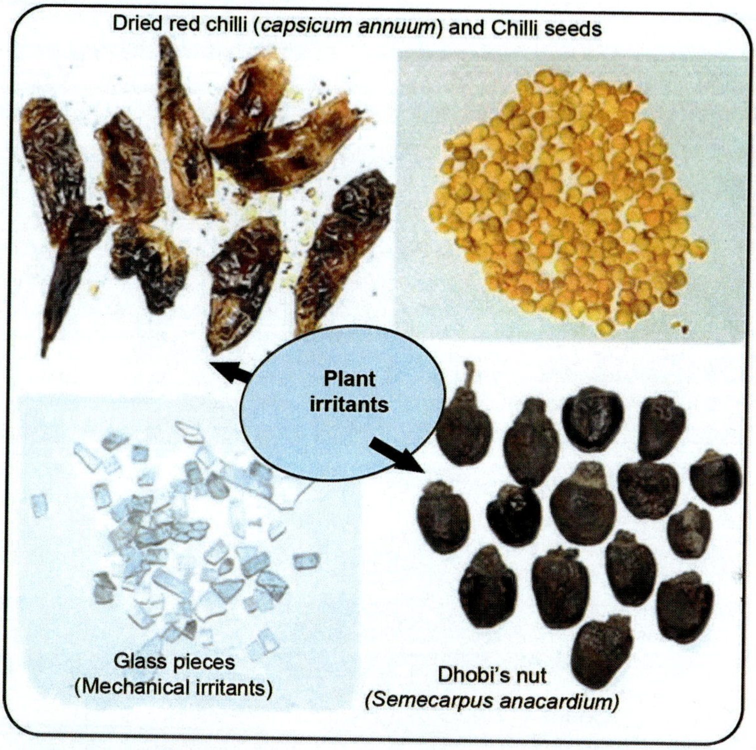
Dried red chilli (capsicum annuum) and Chilli seeds
Plant irritants
Glass pieces (Mechanical irritants)
Dhobi's nut (Semecarpus anacardium)

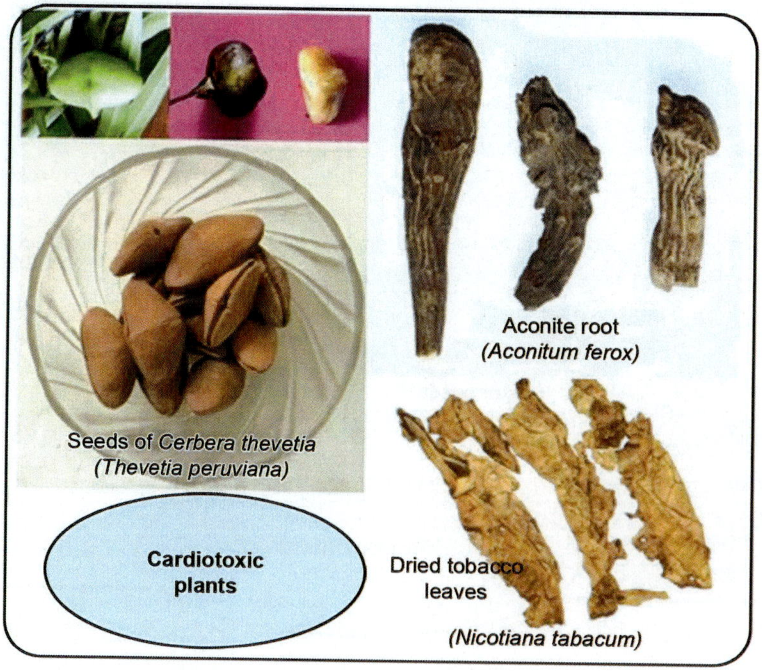
Aconite root (Aconitum ferox)
Seeds of Cerbera thevetia (Thevetia peruviana)
Cardiotoxic plants
Dried tobacco leaves
(Nicotiana tabacum)

Contd...

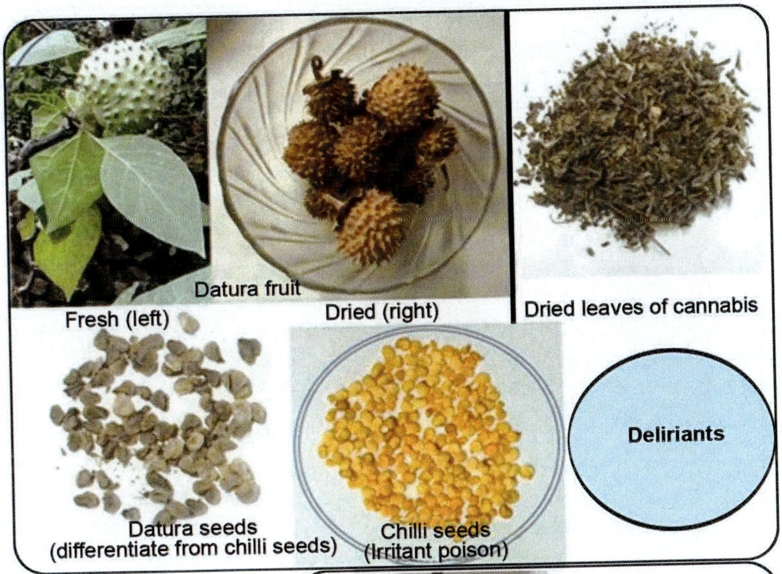
Datura fruit
Fresh (left)
Dried (right)
Dried leaves of cannabis
Deliriants
Datura seeds
(differentiate from chilli seeds)
Chilli seeds
(Irritant poison)

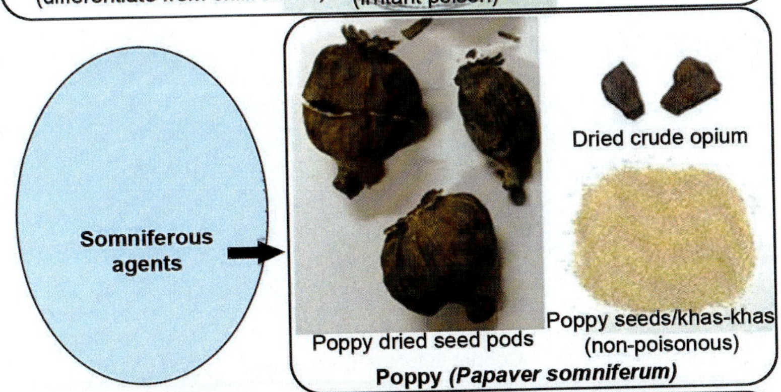
Somniferous agents
Dried crude opium
Poppy dried seed pods
Poppy seeds/khas-khas
(non-poisonous)
Poppy (Papaver somniferum)

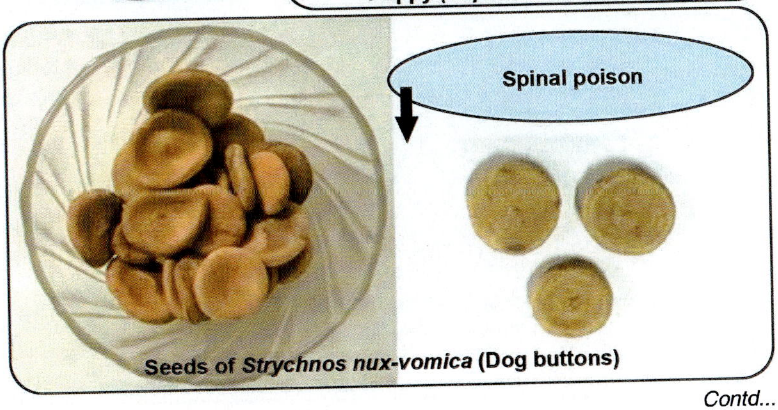
Spinal poison
Seeds of Strychnos nux-vomica (Dog buttons)

Contd...

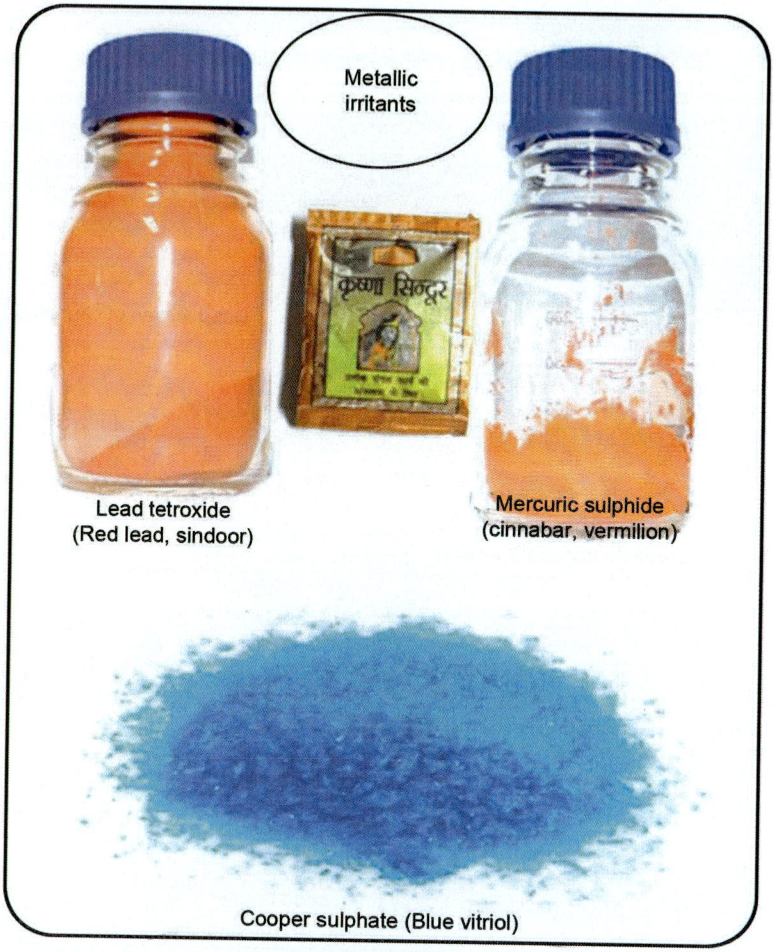
Metallic irritants
कृष्णा सिन्दूर
Lead tetroxide
(Red lead, sindoor)
Mercuric sulphide
(cinnabar, vermilion)
Cooper sulphate (Blue vitriol)

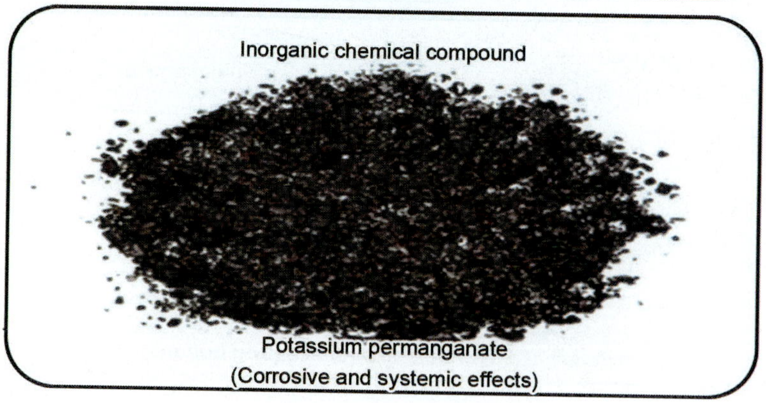
Inorganic chemical compound
Potassium permanganate
(Corrosive and systemic effects)

Contd...

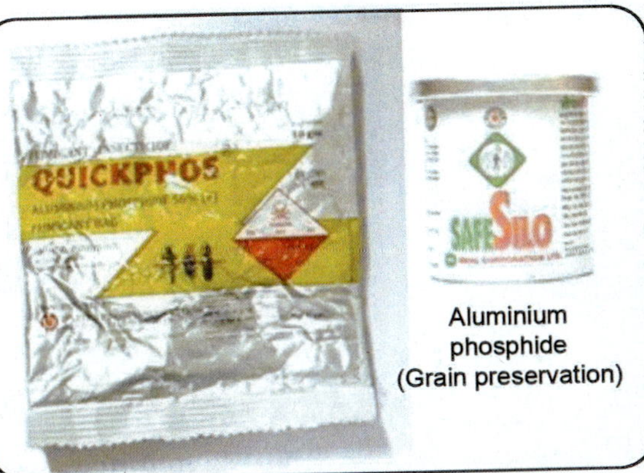

Aluminium phosphide (Grain preservation)

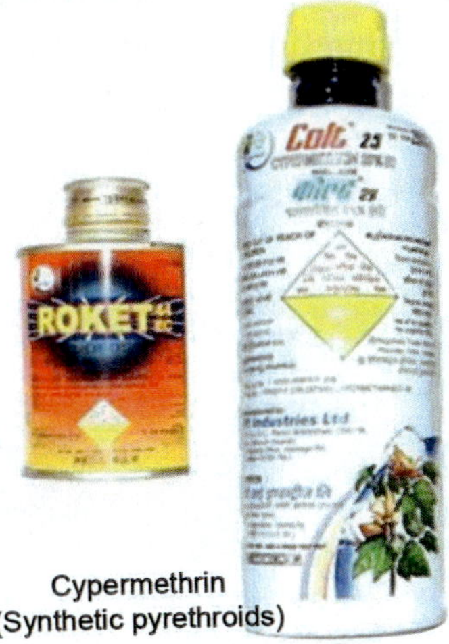

Cypermethrin (Synthetic pyrethroids)

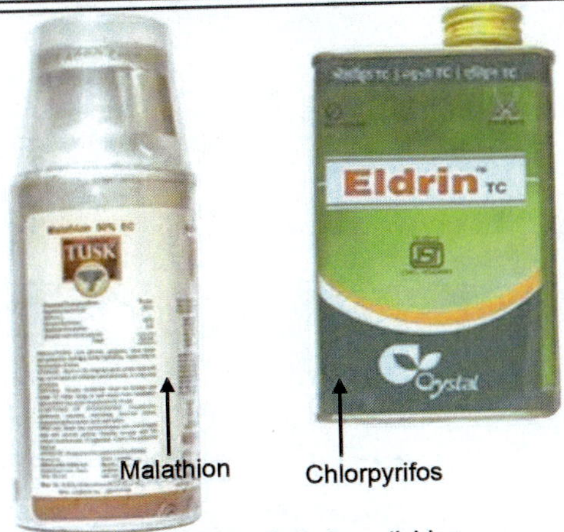

Malathion

Chlorpyrifos

Organophosphate insecticides

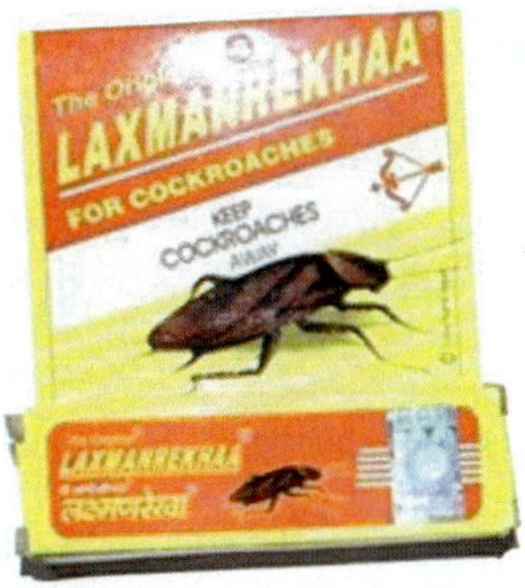

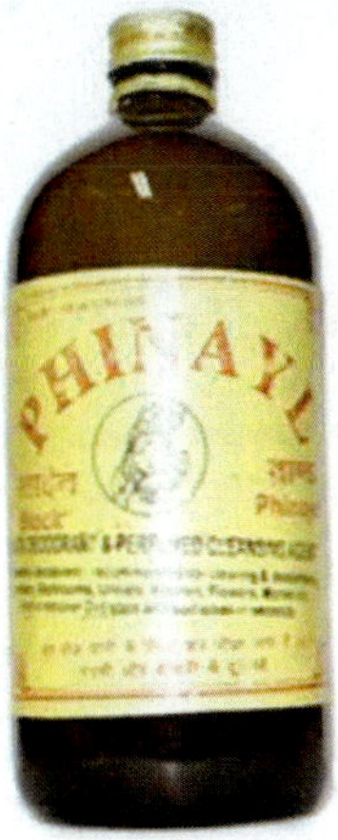

Phenol/Carbolic acid (Corrosive agent)

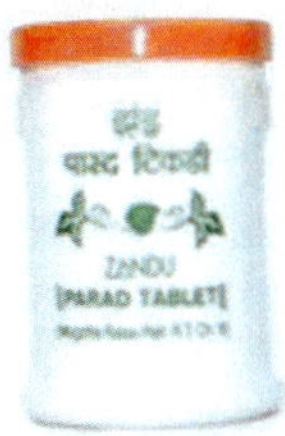

Parad tablet (mercury + chalk)

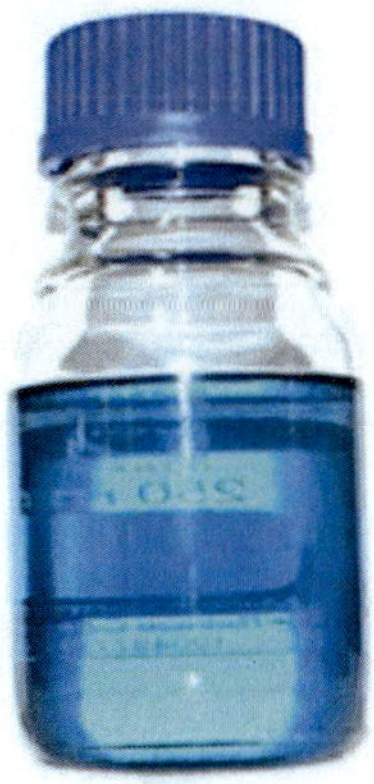

Kerosene

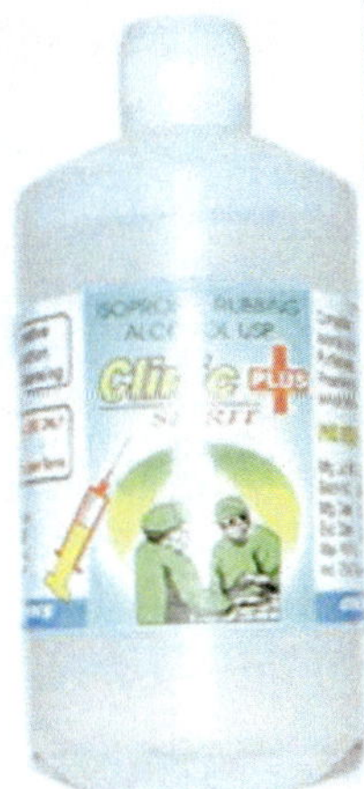

Hand wash (Isopropyl alcohol)

Venomous and Nonvenomous snakes

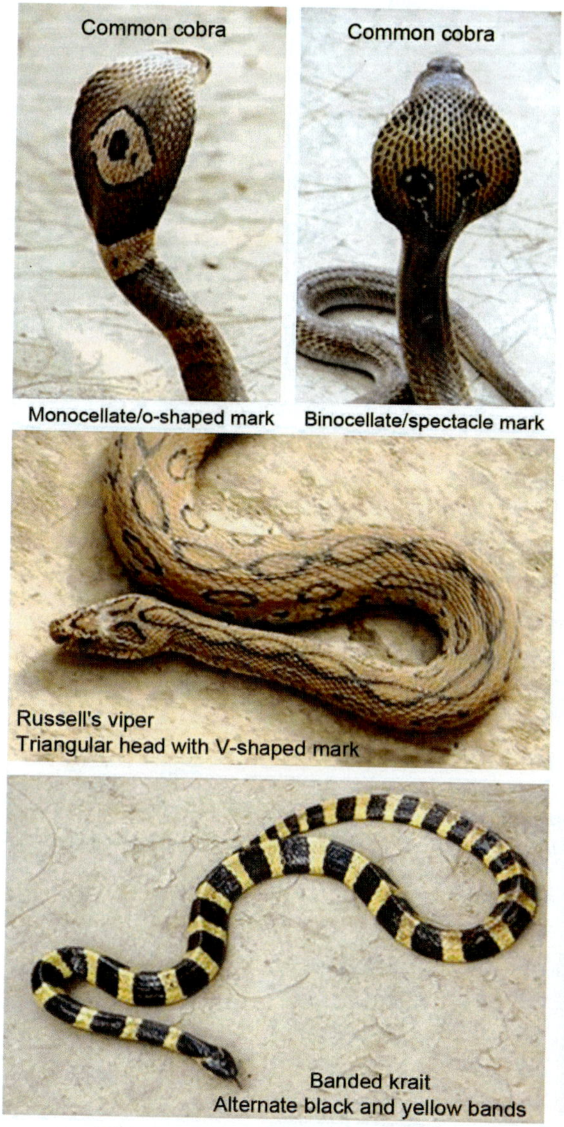

Common venomous snakes in india

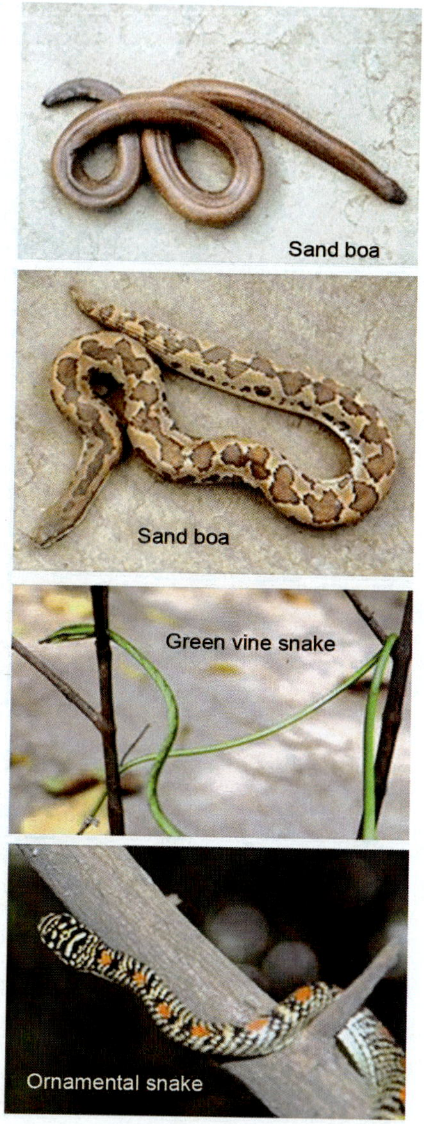

Non-venomous snakes

Pictures credit

Dr Sanjoy Das
Professor and Head
Department of Forensic Medicine and Toxicology
Himalayan Institute of Medical Sciences
Swami Rama Himalayan University
Swami Ram Nagar, Jolly Grant, Dehradun, Uttarakhand.

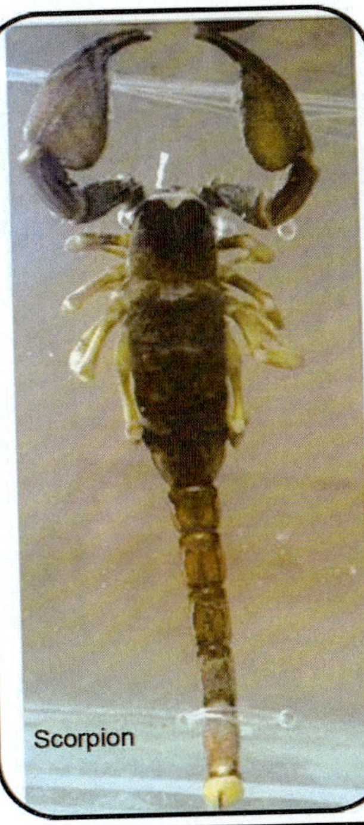

Scorpion

Inebriants

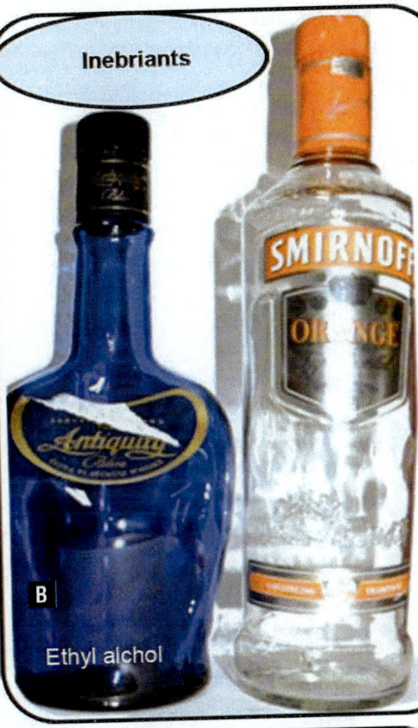

Ethyl alchol

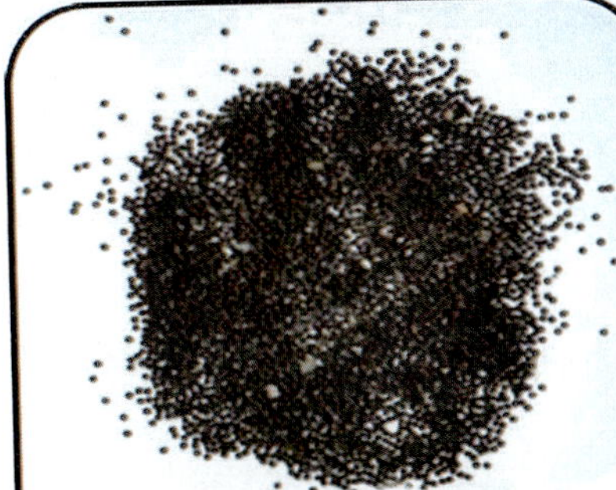

Argemone mexicana
(used as adulterant)

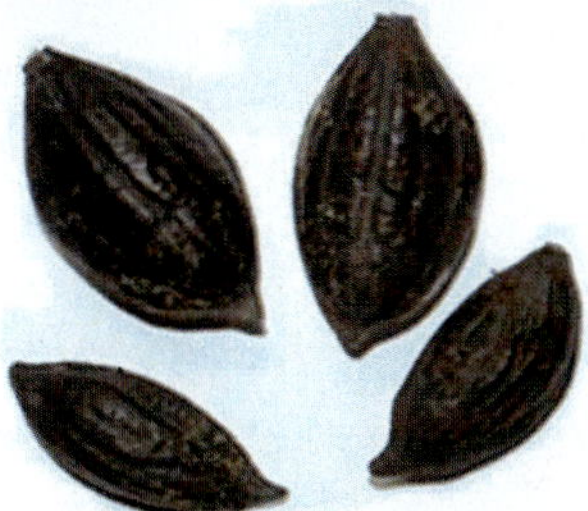

Almonds
(contains cyanide in form of cyanogenic glycoside)

Polyvalent snake venom antiserum

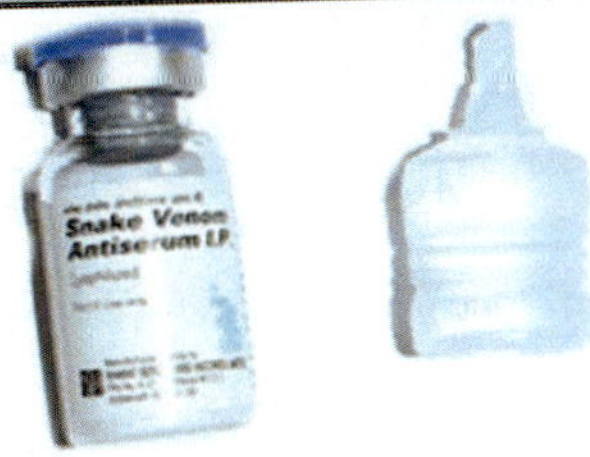

Index

Page numbers followed by *f* refer to figure and *t* refer to table

B

D

E

H

I

K

L